GET THE LOWDOWN
HIGH BLOOD

W9-BJK-535

This guide from the editors of *Prevention* Health Books offers the information and advice you need to take control of your blood pressure *now*. High blood pressure is a silent, symptom-less condition that affects some fifty million Americans. Left untreated, it can set the stage for serious complications—including heart disease, stroke, and kidney damage. But you don't need to let it get that far. With a few simple lifestyle changes and a combination of mainstream and alternative remedies, you can lower your blood pressure to a healthy level—and keep it there.

Inside you'll discover:

- What high blood pressure is and how it happens
- Who is most likely to develop high blood pressure and why
- What complications high blood pressure can cause— and why people with diabetes are at special risk
- What isolated systolic hypertension is and why it matters
- What you should look for when buying a home blood pressure monitor
- What you should know about the most common blood pressure–reducing medications—from aspirin to prescription drugs
- How foods, herbs, and supplements can help lower blood pressure—sometimes eliminating the need for drugs!

OUTSMART HIGH BLOOD PRESSURE

PREVENTION'S™
Outsmart
High Blood Pressure

Also by the Editors of *Prevention* Health Books

Outsmart High Cholesterol

Outsmart Arthritis

The Ice Cream Diet

The Peanut Butter Diet

Anti-Aging Secrets

Complementary Cures

Energy Boosters

Pain-Free Living for Seniors

Fat Fighters

Healing Herbs

Natural Remedies for Women

Power Foods

Vitamin Cures

**Available from
St. Martin's Paperbacks**

PREVENTION'S™

Outsmart High Blood Pressure

EXPERT-ENDORSED SOLUTIONS FOR LOWERING BLOOD PRESSURE QUICKLY AND SAFELY

By the Editors of *Prevention* Health Books

St. Martin's Paperbacks

PREVENTION'S OUTSMART HIGH BLOOD PRESSURE

Copyright © 2003 by Rodale Inc.

Prevention is a registered trademark of Rodale Inc.

ISBN: 0-312-98812-5

Printed in the United States of America

Rodale / St. Martin's Paperbacks edition / September 2003

St. Martin's Paperbacks are published by St. Martin's Press, 175 Fifth Avenue, New York, NY 10010.

10 9 8 7 6 5 4 3 2 1

NOTICE

This book is intended as a reference volume only, not as a medical manual. The information presented here is designed to help you make informed decisions about your health. It is not intended as a substitute for any treatment that may have been prescribed by your doctor. If you suspect that you have a medical problem, we urge you to seek competent medical care. If you have not participated in an exercise program regularly or recently, we encourage you to work with your physician to determine the activity level that is best for you.

Mention of specific companies, organizations, or authorities in this book does not imply endorsement by the publisher, nor does mention of specific companies, organizations, or authorities imply that they endorse the book.

Any Internet addresses and telephone numbers provided in this book were accurate at the time the book went to press.

CONTENTS

INTRODUCTION

Some factors that raise your risk for heart attack and stroke are within your control—like your weight, your eating habits, and your activity level. Others can't be changed—like your age, your race, and your family history.

But one factor may be even more insidious than most. While it's within your control, you may not even realize you have it—many people don't. But that doesn't stop it from harming their bodies day after day, minute by minute.

That factor is high blood pressure. It not only contributes to heart disease and stroke—two leading causes of death in the United States—it also can undermine your vision and inflict severe damage on your kidneys.

Since you've picked up this book, chances are that you've already been diagnosed with high blood pressure. Or perhaps you're at risk for the condition, and you want to find out how to avoid it. Either way, you're being proactive about your health. You can feel good about that.

The fact is, many people can bring their blood pressure into a healthy range just by making sensible lifestyle changes—curbing their alcohol consumption, for example, or quitting smoking. Those who need a little extra help can choose from a range of herbs and nutritional supplements with therapeutic compounds known to rein in blood pressure readings. The most severe cases of high blood pressure may require medical intervention, in the form of prescription drugs. They can lower blood pressure levels *fast*.

You'll get essential information about all of these treatment options in the following pages. Along the way, you'll discover:

- What your blood pressure numbers mean
- Why a low-sodium diet may not be appropriate for everyone
- How adding more steps to your day can put a big dent in your blood pressure reading
- Why managing stress is essential to reducing your risk of heart disease
- Which blood pressure medications work best—and why

To produce this book, we've drawn upon the latest reports from the frontlines of scientific research, as well as the expertise of the country's leading heart-health experts and organizations. So you're getting the latest news and the best advice—just what've you've come to expect from *Prevention,* one of America's most trusted sources for health information.

Armed with this knowledge, you can fight back against high blood pressure and prevent more serious complications down the road. What better way to ensure a long, vital life than to take charge of your health *now?*

PREVENTION'S™
Outsmart
High Blood Pressure

PART I

Blood Pressure Basics

CHAPTER ONE

What's the Big Deal about Blood Pressure?

One-quarter of all American adults—about 50 million people—have high blood pressure, also known as hypertension. And according to recent estimates, as many as one-third of them don't even realize it. This means that roughly 16 million people—or the equivalent of the population of Texas—are walking around with a condition that raises their risk of disabling or fatal illness but generally produces no warning signs.

The American Heart Association identifies high blood pressure as the number one modifiable risk factor for stroke. (In other words, it's within your control, at least to some degree.) In fact, if you have high blood pressure, you're seven times more likely to experience a stroke.

You're also three times more likely to develop coronary artery disease, a narrowing of the arteries that supply blood to the heart. And you're six times more likely to experience congestive heart failure, in which your heart can't pump enough blood to satisfy your body's needs.

But high blood pressure doesn't cause damage overnight. It's more insidious than that. As blood surges through your cardiovascular system, it erodes material from the artery walls, much as a river erodes its bed. Immune cells rush in to make the necessary repairs, leaving behind a thick, hard paste. Over time, the paste begins to clog your arteries, forcing your heart to beat even harder to squeeze blood through narrowed openings. This sets the stage for further damage—and increases pressure inside the arteries to boot.

"If your heart had the benefit of pipes the size of the Hudson River, it wouldn't need to pump much to move the blood," explains Peter M. Abel, M.D., director of cardiovascular disease and prevention at the Cardiovascular Institute of the South in Morgan City, Louisiana. "But if it's dealing with arterial openings the size of the lead in a pencil, it's going to need to push pretty hard." The extra workload can cause your heart to enlarge and to struggle with the delivery of blood throughout your body. And that's just the beginning of the potential problems, as you'll see.

The fact that so many Americans remain blind to the health implications of high blood pressure, not to mention their own elevated blood pressure readings, has become a major public health concern. In a survey of 16,000 people published in *The New England Journal of Medicine*, most of the respondents with untreated or uncontrolled high blood pressure reported that they had seen a doctor in the previous year. For whatever reason, the condition just isn't being taken seriously enough. And that's too bad, because reining in high blood pressure now can head off all sorts of trouble down the road.

A VITAL SIGN

Everyone has blood pressure; it's essential to human life. In a nutshell, it's the force exerted by blood against the

---

PREVENTING THE NEXT ONE

When researchers reviewed health information from 1,252 stroke and heart attack survivors, they made a shocking discovery: About half of the people had done nothing to address risk factors like high blood pressure and high cholesterol, which could lead to a second event. Incredibly, 18 percent continued to smoke.

If you've survived a heart attack or stroke, you've been given a rare second chance. By keeping all scheduled checkups, taking any prescribed medications, and making the necessary lifestyle changes, you can reduce your risk of a recurrence—and stick around a good long time.

---

walls of the arteries as it travels throughout the body. Without blood pressure, blood can't deliver necessary oxygen and nutrients to vital organs so that they can keep functioning.

Your blood pressure reading consists of two numbers, read as a fraction. The top number represents *systolic* pressure, or the force of blood as your heart beats; the bottom number, or *diastolic* pressure, reflects the force of blood as your heart relaxes between beats. Doctors measure blood pressure in millimeters of mercury, or mm Hg.

The National Heart, Lung, and Blood Institute defines optimal blood pressure as less than 120/80 mm Hg. High blood pressure begins at 140/90. If your reading falls anywhere between these two benchmarks, you should pay close attention to it. The higher it climbs, the greater the health risks become. (In Chapter 2, we'll talk more about measuring blood pressure, as well as the prehypertension classification of readings between optimal and high.)

One particular form of high blood pressure—isolated systolic hypertension, or ISH—didn't get much attention until recently. Now doctors say that it's cause for concern, too. In ISH, the systolic reading (the top number) is higher than it should be, while the diastolic reading (the bottom number) is fine. ISH appears most common among older Americans; in fact, about 65 percent of people over age 60 with high blood pressure have ISH, according to the National Heart, Lung, and Blood Institute. And in that survey of 16,000 people mentioned earlier, most of the respondents with uncontrolled high blood pressure had ISH.

MYSTERIOUS ORIGINS

High blood pressure can result from any number of factors. But according to the American Heart Association, doctors are able to pinpoint an exact cause—such as an abnormality in the kidneys or a structural defect in the aorta (the large artery that carries blood from the heart)—in only 5 to 10 percent of cases.

So what's behind all the rest of those cases?

Well, smoking is a major offender, as the nicotine in cigarettes constricts arteries. And a lifetime of eating high-fat foods can cause trouble by raising blood cholesterol, which in turn leads to plaque buildup and narrowed arterial openings.

A high-fat diet also can contribute to weight gain, which itself is a risk factor for high blood pressure. In this country, overweight and obesity have reached epidemic proportions, with more than half of American adults carrying too many pounds.

Imagine what would happen if a pump designed to supply water for a modest single-family home instead were hooked up to an entire condominium complex.

That's pretty much what happens when the heart has to contend with extra body weight. "Fat is alive, and it's very vascular. It needs blood," Dr. Abel explains. "So carrying extra fat makes the heart do extra work."

But even if you weigh exactly what you should, you may find your blood pressure creeping upward as you get older. That's because your arteries naturally become more rigid with age, so your heart must beat harder to sustain bloodflow.

KNOW YOUR RISK

If high blood pressure has a bright side, it's that many risk factors—like overweight and obesity, poor diet, and smoking, as well as an inactive lifestyle and excessive alcohol consumption—are controllable. In other words, you can do something about them.

That said, certain segments of the population are especially susceptible to high blood pressure, often for reasons beyond their control. If you fall into any of the following groups, you and your doctor need to keep close tabs on your blood pressure reading—and to take action as soon as it starts creeping toward "high."

Older people. As mentioned above, the risk of high blood pressure creeps upward with age. Typically, the onset of the condition occurs between ages 35 and 55 in men, and at menopause in women. About 60 percent of all Americans age 60 and older have high blood pressure.

Pregnant women. In the United States, about 7 percent of all mothers-to-be develop blood pressure problems during their pregnancies. Statistics from the National Institutes of Health show that the incidence of preeclampsia, a condition characterized by a sudden rise in blood pressure, has increased by nearly one-third over the past decade. Typically, preeclampsia begins after the 20th week of pregnancy. Left untreated, it can affect the mother's kidneys, liver, and brain. It also is a leading cause of complications such as low birth weight, premature birth, and stillbirth.

African-Americans. High blood pressure affects about one in three African-Americans, a much higher incidence than in whites. What's more, it tends to show up much earlier in life and usually is much more severe, leading to a greater number of deaths from stroke and kidney disease.

People with family histories. If a close blood relative—a parent or a sibling, for example—has high blood pressure, you're more likely to get it, too.

THE PHYSICAL TOLL

Because high blood pressure produces virtually no symptoms, it's easy to ignore. But that doesn't mean it isn't causing harm. In fact, it can do a real number on your arteries, beyond triggering the cascade of events that ultimately narrows arterial openings. It also speeds hardening of the arteries, a condition known as arteriosclerosis.

The trouble is, blood doesn't travel all that well through stiff, inflexible arteries. So the body's vital organs—which rely on blood for oxygen and nutrients—aren't able to perform up to par. Even worse, a blood clot can lodge in a thickened artery, effectively cutting off the blood supply.

In these ways, high blood pressure can help set the stage for a host of serious health problems, including the following:

Heart attack. Your heart muscle needs oxygen in order to keep pumping blood to the rest of your body. If

IS IT A HEART ATTACK?

Each year, about 1.1 million Americans have heart attacks. Of these cases, about 460,000 are fatal, according to the National Institutes of Health.

A heart attack occurs when a blood clot cuts off most or all of the blood supply to the heart. According to the American Heart Association, warning signs of an attack include the following:

• Discomfort in the center of the chest that may feel like pressure, squeezing, fullness, or pain; it can last for several minutes, or disappear and reappear

• Discomfort in one or both arms or the stomach, neck, or jaw

• Shortness of breath, a cold sweat, light-headedness, or nausea

If you think you're having a heart attack, call 911 or your local emergency response number immediately. The sooner doctors can begin testing and treatment, the greater your chance of minimizing damage to your heart.

one of the arteries that feed your heart hardens or narrows, it can slow the flow of oxygen-rich blood to the organ, causing chest pain (also called angina). The total blockage of an artery can result in a heart attack.

Stroke. Most strokes occur when a blood clot forms somewhere in the body and finds its way into an artery that feeds the brain, shutting off bloodflow. Less frequently, an artery actually leaks into the brain, causing a hemorrhage. Between 40 and 90 percent of all stroke patients had high blood pressure prior to their attacks, according to the National Stroke Association.

Kidney damage. Your kidneys play a crucial role in filtering waste from your blood. Given enough time, high blood pressure can narrow and thicken the blood vessels in your kidneys. This impairs the kidneys' function, so they don't eliminate waste as they should. Ultimately, they could fail altogether, leaving dialysis and possibly a kidney transplant as your only treatment options.

Eye damage. High blood pressure can thicken tiny blood vessels in the part of the eye called the retina. Sometimes the vessels become blocked or start bleeding. You might not notice any visual effects at first. But in later stages of the condition (called hypertensive retinopathy), the retina and the optic nerve may swell, leading to diminished vision.

Reproductive damage. In men, the hardening of the arteries caused by high blood pressure can reduce blood-flow to the penis, impairing the ability to have an erection. Long known as impotence, this condition now goes by a more politically correct name: erectile dysfunction.

TAKE ACTION NOW

As you can see, the consequences of untreated or uncontrolled high blood pressure can be quite serious. But they're not inevitable. In many cases, they're completely avoidable. And the sooner you take steps to improve your blood pressure reading, the less likely you are to experience any adverse effects.

For proof, consider the results of a 12-year study that tracked a group of Pittsburgh residents with high blood pressure. Those who sought treatment at the earliest signs of trouble were able to prevent the onset of heart disease, or at least postpone it. On the other hand, those who didn't tend to their high blood pressure early on were three times more likely to develop heart disease or suffer a stroke.

"The people in the study had isolated systolic hypertension [a high top number in a blood pressure reading],"

HYPERTENSION IN HISTORY

The warning signs certainly were there. Just before the invasion of Normandy in June 1944, President Franklin D. Roosevelt's blood pressure was recorded at 226/118. And before the Yalta Conference in February 1945, it was measured at 260/150, according to the personal notes of Howard G. Bruenn, M.D., the cardiologist who cared for FDR during the last year of his life.

But back in the 1940s, not all doctors considered high blood pressure a health risk. In fact, up until the day of his death, FDR's personal physician, Vice Admiral Ross T. McIntire, declared the president to be in excellent health. In reality, the president's blood pressure was eroding his artery walls and enlarging his heart, according to British physician and author Richard Gordon, in his book *An Alarming History of Famous (and Difficult!) Patients*.

What FDR's personal doctors and the rest of America couldn't see, doctors in other parts of the world could, according to Gordon. When Roosevelt went to Yalta, Lord Moran—Winston Churchill's physician—took one look at the president, realized what a sick man he was, and predicted he would not live longer than a few months.

Moran was right. On April 12, 1945, the president complained of a severe headache and lost consciousness immediately afterward. His blood pressure was 300/190 when Dr. Bruenn checked it 15 minutes later. At 3:35 P.M., Roosevelt died of a cerebral hemorrhage.

No autopsy was done to chronicle the extent of FDR's illness. But his arteries were so clogged that during the embalming process, the formaldehyde pump strained and stopped numerous times.

Since the 1940s, modern medicine has made fatal hypertension, as observed in Roosevelt, a rare occurrence.

SPECIAL NEWS FOR DIABETICS

If you've been diagnosed with diabetes, you have even more reason to rein in your blood pressure.

In a survey of more than 1,500 adults with diabetes, more than 70 percent also had high blood pressure. That's nearly three times the incidence among those without diabetes, according to the Centers for Disease Control and Prevention (CDC) in Atlanta. What's more, even though 57 percent of the survey participants were taking blood pressure medication, less than half of them had successfully lowered their blood pressure to a healthy level.

High blood pressure is an especially serious health concern for people with diabetes, because it raises the risk of heart disease, stroke, kidney failure, and vision loss, says researcher Linda S. Geiss, chief of the CDC's diabetes surveillance section. "People with diabetes should make certain that their blood pressure is checked at every doctor's visit," she says.

notes researcher Kim Sutton-Tyrrell, Dr.P.H., of the University of Pittsburgh. "Physicians and patients have been ignoring this condition, even though research has shown that early treatment can save lives."

One of the recommendations to come out of the study is to check your blood pressure at least once a year. If you have a reading of 120/80—what the experts now define as prehypertension—or above, you should go for rechecks two or three times a year.

If you already have high blood pressure (140/90 or above), your doctor should perform a complete physical to assess your risk for the sorts of complications described earlier in the chapter. This information will help determine your treatment protocol. These days, many physicians favor lifestyle strategies—such as losing weight, following a low-sodium diet, and increasing physical activity—as the first-line treatment for all but the most serious blood pressure problems. That said, if your blood pressure remains high after six months despite lifestyle changes, you may need to go on medication.

Through the rest of this book, you'll learn about the full spectrum of approaches to outsmarting high blood pressure, from mainstream medicine to alternative therapies. While the majority of these approaches are ideal for self-care, we still recommend working closely with your doctor. Together, the two of you can devise a plan that effectively lowers your blood pressure without significantly impacting your lifestyle.

After all, for your plan to work, you need to be able to stick with it. Our goal is to make that as easy as possible. Your goal is to succeed!

CHAPTER TWO

Making Sense of the Numbers

Compared with many other medical tests, a blood pressure screening is a breeze. It's quick and painless—and, as a bonus, you get to stay fully clothed.

If you have high blood pressure, you likely will be scheduled for regular screenings at your health care provider's office. Depending on the circumstances, you may be asked to monitor your blood pressure at home as well.

In either case, the better you understand the screening process, the more you'll get from it. It's a vital component of any plan to return your blood pressure to a healthy level.

So consider this chapter your primer on blood pressure screenings. You'll learn how monitors work, what the results mean, and—most important—whether they're accurate. You can use this information to be more proactive in your blood pressure care.

WHAT TO EXPECT FROM A SCREENING

In medical circles, the device that measures your blood pressure goes by the name *sphygmomanometer* (pronounced "sfig-mo-ma-*nohm*-e-ter"). If you've had even one blood pressure screening, you probably know the procedure for using this device by heart (pardon the pun!).

First, the person who's checking your blood pressure—most likely a doctor or a nurse—squeezes a lemon-shaped bulb that pumps air through a tube into an inflatable cuff around your upper arm. The cuff compresses a large artery that runs down your arm, briefly interrupting bloodflow. At that point, the person places a stethoscope over the artery in the vicinity of your inner elbow and turns a valve to slowly release air from the cuff. Then she listens for your pulse.

As blood rushes through the artery, it produces a thumping sound that indicates your systolic pressure, or the top number in your blood pressure reading. Then the sound goes silent, as the pressure in the artery exceeds the pressure in the cuff. This indicates your diastolic pressure—the bottom number. Both numbers appear on a dial or a column of mercury that's connected to the blood pressure monitor.

Not all monitors are the same, of course. Newer models may have electronic instrumentation or digital readouts. Some don't require a stethoscope.

Keep in mind, too, that one reading in the high range—140/90 or above—doesn't mean that you actually have high blood pressure. Some people are prone to what's known as white-coat hypertension. As the name suggests, their blood pressure registers as high only when they're in a doctor's office.

In fact, everyone's blood pressure constantly fluctuates a little. Stress can raise it, as can talking. So can drinking a caffeinated beverage two hours before a screening. Sometimes readings can be higher in the morning than in the afternoon or evening.

FOR GOOD MEASURE

You can take steps to ensure that your blood pressure screening produces an accurate reading. The National Heart, Lung,
and Blood Institute recommends the following:
• Wear short sleeves to expose your arm. A sleeve that's tightly
rolled up could skew your reading.
• Avoid coffee or cigarettes for at least 30 minutes before your
screening.
• For 5 minutes before your screening, sit with your back supported and your feet flat on the ground. Rest your arm on a
table at the level of your heart.
• Go to the restroom before your screening. A full bladder
could affect your reading.
• Ask the doctor or nurse to take two readings at least 2
minutes apart, then average them.
• Be sure to find out your reading in numbers—not just a category such as "normal" or "high."

This is why most health care providers will want to
check your blood pressure several times over the course
of several days before deeming it "high." So if one of
your readings comes in on the high side, don't panic. (It
could skew your blood pressure even more!)

YOUR GUIDE TO HOME MONITORS

Depending on the circumstances, your doctor may recommend keeping a blood pressure monitor at home, so
you can check your own blood pressure periodically.
That way, you can get accurate readings in familiar,
comfortable surroundings. And if you maintain a log of
your readings, your doctor can get a better picture of

your changing blood pressure over time, according to the American Heart Association.

When you're checking your own blood pressure, your best bet is to take two or three readings, especially if you're just learning how to operate the monitor. Also, your doctor may recommend that you check your blood pressure frequently when you're first diagnosed with high blood pressure or you make changes to your treatment regimen. Once you have control of your blood pressure, however, you should be able to cut back on your screenings to once every two weeks, or even once a month, according to the American Medical Association (AMA).

These days, you can buy home blood pressure monitors in drugstores, department stores, and medical supply stores. But be forewarned. The array of models and special features can be mind-boggling. To help with your decision, the American Heart Association has analyzed several of the most popular monitors and identified the pros and cons of each. Here's a quick rundown.

Mercury sphygmomanometer. This is the standard blood pressure monitor. It's durable, it doesn't require readjustment, and it can last a lifetime with minimal maintenance. Home models come with a D-ring cuff and attached stethoscope for convenience and ease of use.

Be aware, though, that the monitors can be quite bulky. And, as their name implies, they do contain mercury, which can be hazardous if it's spilled. To ensure accurate blood pressure readings, the monitors must be kept upright on a flat surface. If you have trouble with your vision or hearing, or if you can't squeeze the pump to inflate the cuff, you may not be able to operate this kind of monitor.

Aneroid sphygmomanometer. Compared with the mercury monitor, the aneroid monitor tends to be less expensive, more lightweight, and more portable. The gauge works in any position. Some models are equipped with especially easy-to-read gauges, as well as D-ring cuffs for one-handed use and built-in or attached stethoscopes.

If the monitors have a downside, it's that they contain delicate, easily damaged internal mechanisms. For this reason, they need to be checked against a mercury monitor at least once a year, or whenever they're jarred. Like the mercury monitor, the aneroid monitor may be not be suitable for people who don't see or hear well, or who have difficulty squeezing the pump to inflate the cuff.

Automatic sphygmomanometer. With this kind of monitor, all the components are housed in one unit, which isn't as cumbersome as a separate gauge and stethoscope. Most models are portable and easy to operate, with a D-ring cuff for one-handed use. In addition, some higher-end models offer automatic inflation and deflation, digital readouts, and a print function to record your readings on paper. The automatic monitors are ideal for people with impaired vision or hearing.

Unfortunately, the monitors don't provide accurate readings for everyone. You need to make sure that the cuff is properly positioned on your arm or wrist, or else the monitor may not work. And if you happen to need a larger cuff, you may have a hard time finding one. Like the aneroid monitors, the automatic monitors come with complex, fragile internal mechanisms. They need to be checked against a mercury monitor on a regular basis.

Now, you may be wondering about those blood pressure screening machines that have been popping up in drugstores and supermarkets. While they're okay for occasional use, the American Medical Association cautions

CUFF SIZE MATTERS

If you're thinking of getting a home blood pressure monitor, be sure to choose one with the proper cuff size. It can affect the accuracy of your reading, according to the American Medical Association (AMA).

The AMA recommends using a cuff that's wide enough to reach from just below your armpit to the inside of your elbow. It should go completely around your arm with a few inches to spare.

In general, you'll need a small cuff (5 × 9 inches) if the distance from your shoulder to your elbow is less than 13 inches. If it's between 13 and 16 inches, get a medium cuff (6 × 13 inches). More than 16 inches requires a large cuff (7 × 14 inches).

against relying on them as a substitute for checking your blood pressure with a sphygmomanometer. They're sensitive to hand and arm movement, which cuts down on their accuracy. That said, if you consistently get high readings from these machines, you should see your doctor for a follow-up screening.

WHAT YOUR READING MEANS

As explained in Chapter 1, a blood pressure reading of less than 120/80 qualifies as optimal, while a reading of 140/90 or above is considered high. But what if yours falls between the two extremes? Then you have prehypertension, according to the newly revised guidelines of the National Heart, Lung, and Blood Institute.

If the top and bottom numbers of your blood pressure reading fall into two different categories, you should go with the higher one in assessing your blood pressure level. A reading of 130/70, for example, would constitute prehypertension.

Incidentally, if you have a prehypersensitive reading, please don't ignore it. Even though it's not quite as serious as high blood pressure, it could lead to major problems if it isn't taken care of.

In a report published in the British medical journal *Lancet*, researchers involved in the long-running Framingham Heart Study found that nearly 40 percent of people under age 65 with high-normal blood pressure—previously defined as a reading between 130/85 and 139/89—developed high blood pressure within four years. The risk was even greater for people age 65 and older. By comparison, only 18 percent of those with normal blood pressure ended up with high blood pressure.

For a separate report, the same team of researchers determined that over a 10-year period, 4 percent of women and 8 percent of men under age 65 with high-normal blood pressure experienced a heart attack or stroke, developed congestive heart failure, or died from cardiovascular disease. For people age 65 and older, those figures climbed to 18 percent of women and 25 percent of men.

Based on these findings, the experts behind the *Harvard Health Letter* concluded that people with high-normal blood pressure "shouldn't necessarily feel that this is a safe pressure." They recommended strategies such as building meals around plant foods, cutting back on salt and alcohol, increasing physical activity, and maintaining a healthy weight. Together these strategies can help lower your blood pressure to an optimal level.

HOW LOW CAN YOU GO?

In general, people become concerned about their blood pressure only when it's too high. But you can have a reading that's too *low*, which could lead to symptoms like light-headedness and fainting.

Some people appear more prone to low blood pressure than others. For example, it may be more common in those with nervous system disorders, such as diabetic neuropathy, and endocrine disorders, such as parathyroid disease. It also can occur with certain medications, extended bed rest, excessive bleeding, and shock. Other possible factors include overly aggressive treatment of high blood pressure, a faulty heart valve or serious disruption of heart rhythm, or an allergic reaction known as anaphylaxis.

As you can see, almost all of these are potentially serious health concerns. That's why experts advise people with consistently low blood pressure to undergo appropriate testing to rule out an underlying medical cause.

If you feel faint when you stand up, you may have a particular form of low blood pressure called orthostatic hypotension. It happens as blood tries to pool in your legs, the result of gravity. Normally, the body compensates by constricting blood vessels and increasing the heart rate, according to experts at the Mayo Clinic. But in orthostatic hypotension, this corrective mechanism doesn't function as it should.

To diagnose the condition, your doctor likely will recommend what's known as a tilt-table test. During the test, technicians track your blood pressure and heart rate while you lie on a table that moves from a horizontal position to vertical.

PART II

Lifestyle Strategies for Lower Blood Pressure

CHAPTER THREE

Ramp Up Your Activity Level

We have some great news about achieving and maintaining healthy blood pressure. But first . . . are you sitting down? If so, perhaps you shouldn't be.

Physical activity can play an important role in preventing or reversing high blood pressure. In fact, studies show that men and women who are sedentary have a 20 to 50 percent greater risk of developing high blood pressure than those who are physically active.

But the good news is, once you start exercising, you'll notice the benefits almost immediately. When researchers at the University of Pittsburgh instructed 12 overweight women to ride a stationary bike or walk for an hour a day, their blood pressure fell 4 points in just a week.

How does exercise help? By relaxing and dilating the blood vessels so that they're wide open. This reduces the workload on the heart, which doesn't have to pump as hard to move blood throughout the body.

Of course, a regular fitness program also helps melt away any extra pounds, another important factor for controlling blood pressure. Actually, losing as few as 10 pounds can shave points from a blood pressure reading, with the greatest reductions occurring in people who are overweight and already have high blood pressure.

EVERY MOVE MATTERS

According to the American College of Sports Medicine (ACSM), most people with high blood pressure have only a mild to moderate problem. In such cases, three to six months of increased physical activity—combined with a reduced salt intake and effective weight management—are the ideal first-line treatment.

Even for those with more severe high blood pressure, the one-two punch of regular exercise and prescription medication can produce even bigger reductions in blood pressure. In fact, with exercise, people may not need as much medication to begin with.

In general, the ACSM says, raising your activity level can lower your systolic and diastolic blood pressure readings by about 10 points in just three to four weeks. And exercise offers many other health benefits besides. In particular, it gets rid of excess body weight *and* helps control cholesterol and blood sugar—all of which add up to a diminished risk of heart disease and diabetes.

We're not talking about Olympic-caliber workouts either. It's the everyday activities—the stroll from the car to the office, the quick 10-minute walk after lunch, the trip to the corner mailbox to drop a letter—that make a big difference. That's right: just taking a few more steps over the course of a day can lead to healthier blood pressure, which means better protection against heart disease and stroke.

In a study published in the journal *Medicine and Science in Sports and Exercise*, fifteen postmenopausal women with high blood pressure made small changes in their daily routines to increase their daily "mileage" by 4,000 to 5,000 steps. The results: six of the women lowered their blood pressure to a normal level, while another three dropped to borderline normal. The average reduction was 11 points.

But here's the kicker: The women—who hadn't been working out regularly before the study—usually logged their extra steps simply by building more short walks into their days. They parked their cars farther away from the supermarket or the workplace, used the stairs instead of the elevator, or took a few laps around the mall before doing their shopping. They wore lightweight clip-on pedometers to keep track of their mileage.

"Any physical activity can help lower blood pressure, but we chose walking because it's so easy," explains Kerrie L. Moreau, Ph.D., a research associate at the University of Colorado in Boulder. She believes that it can be of just as much benefit to men as to the women in the study.

But you don't have to walk if you don't want to. What matters most is that you're moving—whether you're pedaling your bike or painting your house, rowing a boat or mowing the lawn. The National Heart, Lung, and Blood Institute recommends 30 minutes of moderate physical activity most days, if not every day, to help control blood pressure. How you spend those 30 minutes really is up to you (though we'll offer a few ideas a bit later in the chapter).

STRATEGIES FOR SUCCESS

If you've been relatively sedentary, the first steps of your exercise program will be the toughest. But don't give up! With a little time, your workouts will become second nature. These tips can help you start on the right foot—and stick with it.

Talk with your doctor. Before you launch your exercise program, be sure to get your doctor's okay. He may recommend checking your blood pressure before and after your workouts. (To learn more about home blood pressure monitors, see Chapter 2.) If you notice any sharp increases or drops in your readings, bring them to your doctor's attention. You may need to make some adjustments in your routine so that it's better suited to your fitness level.

Heed the warning signs. If you experience headaches, faintness, or excessive perspiration during your workouts, slow down and check your heart rate. It should fall in the range of 130 to 140 beats per minute. If it's higher than that, stop exercising and rest until it returns to normal.

Designate your workout days. You should try to exercise at least three to five days a week, especially if you want to lose weight. Your best bet is to pick your days up-front, even blocking out time for your workout sessions in your planner or personal organizer. "If you just say, 'I'm going to exercise three days this week,' it'll never happen," says exercise physiologist Robert Brosmer, vice president of health and wellness at the Central Florida YMCA in Orlando. "But if you plan ahead and mark your calendar, you'll do it."

Ease into it, ease out of it. No matter if you're walking, swimming, or playing racquetball, you must allow time to warm up before your workout and cool down after. "Too many people start pushing themselves as hard as they can as soon as they tie their shoes," says John D. McPhail, senior health educator at the Michigan Public Health Institute in Okemos. "Then after two minutes, they feel awful. They blame it on being in terrible shape, and they quit. All they really need to do is warm up."

When you're ready for your workout, go easy for the first 5 to 10 minutes. Walk at a slow pace. Take some leisurely strokes in the pool. Hit a few volleys on the racquetball court. As your body becomes warmer and more limber, you can increase your intensity.

At the end of your workout, wind down with another 5 to 10 minutes of gentle activity. Stopping abruptly can cause dizziness.

Temper your arm movements. Be careful about doing too much arm pumping during your workouts, advises Gerald Fletcher, M.D., a cardiologist at the Mayo Clinic in Jacksonville, Florida. Vigorous movements—as when using a cross-country ski machine or performing certain steps in an aerobics class—can cause a temporary increase in blood pressure. If you're new to exercise, you may want to avoid these kinds of activities until you're in better shape. Or use just your legs. On a ski machine, for example, you can hold your arms at your sides while you slide your legs forward and back.

Pack your shoes. Life is unpredictable, but your exercise program shouldn't suffer because of it. "Simply take your walking shoes wherever you go," says James Rippe, M.D., associate professor of medicine at Tufts University School of Medicine in Boston and author of *Fit over Forty*. "Whether you're on business or on vacation, you're going to have some downtime when you can get out for an invigorating walk. As long as you have your shoes, you can fit a workout into even the most hectic schedule."

Make fitness a family affair. These days, you can easily include your kids or grandkids in your workouts—whether you're walking, hiking, or biking. "You can buy baby joggers, baby backpacks, off-road strollers, bike seats, and even bike attachments that allow the child to sit in back and pedal, too," McPhail says. "You get a great workout—and you teach your children or grandchildren a healthy way of life."

Set your routine to music. If your workout sometimes feels tiring and tedious—which can happen, especially when you're on a treadmill or a stationary bike—simply add music. "Research shows that when people listen to music while they exercise, they don't feel like they're working hard," Brosmer says. "And they keep at it longer."

Mix up your activities. You may love ice cream, but if you eat the same flavor day after day, you're bound to get sick of it. The same is true for exercise, says certified personal trainer Jana Angelakis, founder of PEx Personalized Exercise in New York City. The walking routine that felt so good when you started can seem stale when you've been at it for a few months. "If you're feeling uninspired, don't blame exercise," Angelakis advises. "Blame boredom. Find a new place to walk, or try a whole new activity. It will invigorate you immediately."

FITNESS FAVORITES

Most experts would agree that the key to sticking with an exercise program is to find an activity you enjoy. "Don't do something you hate just because it's good for you," Angelakis says. "You'll get frustrated and discouraged. When you do something you like, you'll always make time for it, and you'll feel great about it."

Not sure what you like? You're not alone. "When you're just starting out, picking an activity can be confusing," Angelakis says. "Your best bet is to find a few that interest you and then try each on for size."

WHAT HAVE YOU GOT TO LOSE?

If you're wondering whether you ought to lose a few pounds, you may want to calculate your body mass index, or BMI. According to federal government guidelines, the combination of BMI and waist circumference can help determine whether your weight could be raising your risk for health problems, particularly heart disease.

To calculate your BMI, follow these steps.

1. Multiply your weight in pounds by 703.
2. Divide the result by your height in inches.
3. Again divide the result by your height in inches.

The final figure is your BMI. What does it mean?

18.5 to 24.9: Your weight is appropriate for your height. You don't need to slim down.

25.0 to 29.9: Your BMI falls in the overweight category. You definitely should get rid of the extra pounds if you meet *both* of the following criteria:

• You have a waist measurement of more than 35 inches if you're a woman or more than 40 inches if you're a man.

• You have at least two other risk factors for heart disease, such as a personal history of high blood pressure, high cholesterol, diabetes, physical inactivity, or smoking; or a family history of heart disease.

30 or higher: Your BMI is in the obese category. You definitely need to lose weight.

To help you sift through the choices, we've put together brief profiles of the most popular activities. Of course, you should not feel limited to these. Instead, think of them as a jumping-off point. (Please note that the calorie burn for each activity has been calculated for a 150-pound person. It may be a bit higher or lower, depending on your own weight.)

Walking. This is the easiest form of exercise by far.

You just put one foot in front of the other. "It's gentle on your joints," Brosmer notes. "And you can do it absolutely anywhere."

You may want to clip a pedometer to your waistband to track your mileage. You should be able to find one in a sporting goods store. Aim for a total of 10,000 steps a day. In the study mentioned earlier, involving 15 post-menopausal women, they were logging 4,000 to 5,000 steps a day in the course of their normal activities. Their blood pressure declined once they added another 4,000 to 5,000 steps.

That may seem like a lot, but it really isn't. Just look for easy ways to slip a few extra steps into your daily routine, like the women in the study. Use a push mower when you trim your lawn, stand up and pace around while you're talking on the phone, take a lap or two around the perimeter of the supermarket before you start grocery shopping. All those steps add up fast!

What you need: A good pair of walking shoes.

Calories burned: 200 to 400 an hour, depending on your pace.

The price tag: About $70 for the shoes.

Special benefits: Walking is an extremely social activity. "It's easy to find a buddy," McPhail notes. "And almost every community has walking clubs. Check with your local mall, community education office, or park office."

Jogging. Compared with walking, jogging can burn more calories in a shorter amount of time, Brosmer says. But it also is harder on your joints. So skip the pavement and stick with dirt trails and gravel tracks.

What you need: Running shoes.

Calories burned: 500 to 600 an hour at a moderate pace.

The price tag: About $70 for the shoes.

Special benefits: Runner's high. "The psychological benefits of pushing yourself a little bit are real," says Deborah Saint-Phard, M.D., an exercise physiologist for the Women's Sports Medicine Center at the Hospital for Special Surgery in New York City. "All those feel-good hormones (called endorphins) kick in, and you feel great."

Swimming. Exercising in water uses all your major muscles and is great for aerobic conditioning, Brosmer says. Just keep in mind that swimming doesn't heat your body as much as exercising on land, because of the coolness of the water. As a result, it doesn't burn as much fat. So if you're trying to lose weight, you may want to combine swimming with another activity.

What you need: A bathing suit and a place to swim.

Calories burned: 400 to 550 an hour swimming freestyle at a slow to moderate pace.

The price tag: Pool memberships vary in price, but you can swim year-round at your local YMCA for about $25 a month.

Special benefits: Swimming is very easy on the joints, thanks to the buoyancy of the water. Even people who are very overweight find that they feel comfortable exercising in a pool.

Bicycling. Zooming around on your two-wheeler, you can't help feeling like a kid again! Bicycling is invigorating, and, as a bonus, it's easy on your joints.

What you need: A bike and a helmet.

Calories burned: 400 to 550 an hour pedaling at a moderate pace.

The price tag: Approximately $200 and up for a bike, and $30 and up for a helmet.

Special benefits: If you don't feel comfortable riding outside, you can get the same benefits from a stationary bike. Even better, enroll in an indoor Spinning class. Most health clubs offer them.

Dancing. Aside from the great music and the fun, dancing offers a super workout.

What you need: A little space and some good tunes.

Calories burned: About 375 an hour for ballroom, disco, folk, or square dancing; about 200 for the slow, romantic variety.

The price tag: Free at home. Private lessons start at about $25 an hour.

Special benefits: "Dancing isn't just good for your body, it's also good for your soul," Dr. Rippe says. "It's one of the most positive mind-body activities around."

Tennis. Spend an afternoon on the court, volleying with a friend. "You don't even have to keep score," Dr. Saint-Phard says. "Just hit the ball back and forth."

What you need: A tennis racquet, balls, and a court to play on.

Calories burned: About 500 an hour playing singles.

The price tag: About $70 for a racquet and $3 for a can of balls. Community courts are free. If you need lessons, the U.S. Tennis Association sometimes offers free clinics. Check your local newspaper.

Special benefits: Playing tennis is great for your lower body, especially your butt and legs.

Hiking. It may be nothing more than walking on trails. But you get to see beautiful landscapes and enjoy the great outdoors.

What you need: Boots and drinking water.

Calories burned: 400 to 500 an hour at a moderate pace.

The price tag: $75 for boots. No need for a special pack for short dayhikes. Just use a fanny pack to carry your water and snacks.

Special benefits: Hiking provides super toning for your butt and legs.

Inline skating. An updated version of roller skating, inline skating is fast, fun, and easy on the joints. Plus, it can burn as many calories as jogging.

What you need: Skates, helmet, and pads.

Calories burned: 400 to 600 an hour, depending on your pace.

The price tag: Skates and safety equipment can cost about $250. Some sporting goods stores offer free lessons. They also may rent out skates for a day, so you can try them before you buy.

Special benefits: Your kids or grandkids will love it, too.

Aerobics. If the word *aerobics* prompts visions of bouncy twentysomethings in spandex thongs, rest assured: Aerobics classes have come a long way. "Most exercise facilities offer a wide variety of classes for people of all fitness levels," says Michael Bourque, certified personal trainer and personal training coordinator for the Center for Health and Wellness of the Central Florida YMCA in Oviedo. The choices range from traditional low-impact aerobics to high-energy workouts like kickboxing.

What you need: Aerobic or cross-training shoes.

Calories burned: About 450 an hour for a high-impact workout.

The price tag: About $70 for the shoes. Classes at the YMCA cost about $25 a month.

Special benefits: Most aerobics classes have certified instructors, which means you'll be getting expert training to maximize the effectiveness of your workouts and minimize your risk of injury. You also get to meet new people and have a great time.

DON'T FORGET STRENGTH TRAINING

These days, most experts recommend strength training as an important component of any exercise program. While it may not have a direct impact on your blood pressure, it does offer other health benefits that ultimately can shave points from your reading. Namely, it builds lean muscle tissue, which keeps burning calories even when you're at rest. That's because muscle needs lots of calories, as well as oxygen, to sustain itself.

In fact, research has shown that a strength-training session can shift your metabolism into overdrive for about 30 minutes after your workout. The more calories you burn, the more pounds you lose—and that can help rein in your blood pressure.

If you already belong to a gym or health club, you likely have access to an array of free weights and Nautilus machines for your strength training. But you can get an equally effective workout in the comfort of your own home, using some basic gear such as dumbbells or weighted medicine balls.

You don't need to spend hours lifting either. In 20 minutes, two or three days a week, you can hit all of your major muscle groups with a handful of exercises, like the following:

- Half-squats, bending at your knees while holding a weight in each hand at shoulder level
- Chest presses, lying on your back and lowering a pair of weights toward your shoulders from an extended position
- Bent-over rows, leaning forward and pulling a weight toward your chest, one arm at a time
- Biceps curls, standing upright and raising a pair of weights toward your collarbone from your sides
- Triceps kickbacks, leaning forward and pushing a weight

straight behind your body from a bent position, one arm
at a time
- Lateral raises, lifting a pair of weights out to the sides with
your palms facing in
- Crunches, raising your upper body while lying on your back
with your knees bent

If you're new to strength training, we recommend a
few sessions with a personal trainer, who can help put
together a workout and provide instruction in proper lifting technique. A good rule of thumb is to use light
weights and perform lots of repetitions. Most important,
remember to keep breathing when lifting—holding your
breath can elevate your blood pressure.

Upper body exercises also can cause a temporary
spike in your blood pressure, especially if you raise your
arms above your head. Try to keep your arms at or below
the level of your heart. Also steer clear of exercises such
as the incline crunch, during which your head is lower
than your heart.

CHAPTER FOUR

Fine-Tune Your Eating Habits

If you've been diagnosed with high blood pressure, your doctor probably has recommended dietary changes as either a first-line treatment or a companion to prescription medication. And for good reason: Research has shown that eating more of some foods and less of others can help lower blood pressure by attacking it on several fronts. That's why a sensible, nutritious diet is an essential component of any blood pressure–management plan.

"High blood pressure is a reflection of a cardiovascular system that's about to burst internally," notes John A. McDougall, M.D., medical director of the McDougall Program at St. Helena Hospital in Napa Valley, California, and author of *The McDougall Program for a Healthy Heart.* "But if you eat a good diet—lots of fruits and vegetables and starch-based foods, versus rich foods—you can help change all that."

Eating a good diet has another important benefit: It pares down your shape. Shedding just 5 to 10 pounds can chip points from your blood pressure reading. What's the connection between overweight and high blood pressure? The more tissue you have on your body, the harder your heart must pump to nourish it. That extra work leads to greater pressure on your artery walls.

Conveniently enough, the same dietary approach recommended for controlling blood pressure—emphasizing low-fat foods, especially fruits and vegetables—also works for whittling your waistline. "This sort of diet is almost certain to lower your blood pressure, because it reduces sodium while increasing the good stuff, like fiber, calcium, and potassium," says Pao-Hwa Lin, Ph.D., director of the clinical nutrition research unit at the Sarah W. Stedman Center for Nutritional Studies at Duke University Medical Center in Durham, North Carolina. "It also is an effective avenue to weight loss."

With its focus on low-fat foods, this sort of diet won't allow for large amounts of red meat, which is loaded with saturated fat. Nor will it accommodate many processed foods. They not only are high in fat but also contain lots of sodium and little potassium. Get rid of them, and you wipe out three dietary bad birds with one stone.

DASH TO HEALTHIER BLOOD PRESSURE

The National Heart, Lung, and Blood Institute recommends an eating plan that adheres to the same core principles described above. The plan goes by the name DASH, for Dietary Approaches to Stop Hypertension. It is considered one of the most effective measures for keeping blood pressure in a healthful range. In fact, it's so effective that people who have followed it have been able to reduce their blood pressure as much as if they had been taking prescription drugs.

In a nutshell, the DASH diet calls for the following:

• Eight to ten servings of fruits and vegetables a day (one serving equals about ½ cup)

- Seven or eight servings of whole grains a day (one serving equals one slice of bread or about ½ cup cooked rice, pasta, or cereal)
- Two or three servings of low-fat or fat-free dairy products a day (one serving equals 1 cup yogurt or milk, or 1 ½ ounces cheese)
- Two or fewer servings of lean meat, poultry, or fish a day (one serving equals about 3 ounces)
- Four or five servings of nuts, seeds, and dry beans a week (one serving equals ⅓ cup nuts, ½ ounce seeds, or ½ cup cooked dry beans)
- Two or three servings of fats and oils a day (one serving equals 1 teaspoon vegetable oil or soft margarine)
- Five sweets per week (such as 1 tablespoon sugar or 8 ounces lemonade)

The National Heart, Lung, and Blood Institute created a 7-day menu plan based on the DASH diet guidelines. We'll get into the specifics of the plan in Chapter 8.

In one study, researchers pitted the DASH diet against two other eating plans—one patterned after the typical American diet, the other similar to the typical American diet but with more fruits and vegetables. All three plans supplied about 3,000 milligrams of sodium a day.

Of the 459 adults in the study, 27 percent of whom had high blood pressure, those who followed the DASH diet or the modified American diet with extra fruits and vegetables experienced reductions in blood pressure. But the DASH diet produced better results, especially in the people with high blood pressure. And those results appeared within just 2 weeks.

A separate study, called DASH-Sodium, also tested the DASH diet against an eating plan based on the typical American diet. Only this time, each plan had three sodium levels: high (3,300 milligrams daily), medium

(2,400 milligrams), and low (1,500 milligrams). The 412 people recruited for the study—41 percent of whom had high blood pressure—followed one of the plans at all three sodium levels.

Of the two eating plans, the DASH diet had a greater impact on blood pressure across the board. But the most significant improvement occurred at the 1,500-milligram level. On the version of the DASH diet with that low amount of sodium, people with *and* without high blood pressure saw dramatic declines in their readings.

THE TROUBLE WITH SODIUM

Why is sodium such an issue? Because too much of the mineral can cause the body to retain extra fluid. This extra fluid could make the heart work harder, which in turn could make blood pressure rise.

We say "could," because not everyone responds to sodium in the same way. According to experts at the Mayo Clinic, some people can consume the mineral with minimal effect on their blood pressure, while others— as much as 40 percent of the population with high blood pressure—are quite sensitive to it. Unfortunately, doctors have no simple test for determining who falls into which category.

Under current government dietary guidelines, most Americans can consume up to 2,400 milligrams of sodium a day, which amounts to about a teaspoon of table salt. Several recent studies suggest this cap may be too high. When men and women without high blood pressure cut their daily sodium intakes by about one-third of the recommended limit—to 1,500 milligrams, or a little less than ⅔ teaspoon—their systolic pressure fell by 7 points. Among those with high blood pressure, systolic pressure dropped even more, by 11½ points.

SALT-FREE SEASONINGS

You don't need salt to liven up the flavor of your meals. So set aside the shaker and reach for the spice rack instead. The following herb and spice suggestions come from the folks at the National Heart, Lung, and Blood Institute (who must spend some time in the kitchen, too!).

- Beef: bay leaf, marjoram, nutmeg, onion, pepper, sage, thyme
- Lamb: curry powder, garlic, mint, rosemary
- Pork: garlic, onion, oregano, pepper, sage
- Veal: bay leaf, curry powder, ginger, marjoram, oregano
- Chicken: ginger, marjoram, oregano, paprika, rosemary, sage, tarragon, thyme
- Fish: curry powder, dill, dry mustard, lemon juice, marjoram, paprika, pepper
- Carrots: cinnamon, cloves, nutmeg, rosemary, sage
- Corn: cumin, curry powder, onion, paprika, parsley
- Green beans: curry powder, dill, lemon juice, marjoram, oregano, tarragon, thyme
- Peas: ginger, marjoram, onion, parsley, sage
- Tomatoes: basil, bay leaf, dill, marjoram, onion, oregano, parsley, pepper

Reducing your sodium intake is a bit more complicated than leaving the salt shaker off the dinner table—though that certainly can help! Sodium and salt, or sodium chloride, occur in measurable amounts in a whole host of foods—especially processed ones.

If you already are watching your sodium intake, you probably have been forgoing the salty chips and pretzels. But you still may be getting a good dose of sodium from other, less obvious sources. Dried fruit, for example, contains sodium sulfite. And ice cream may be made with sodium caseinate and sodium alginate.

Even a sharp-eyed sodium detective can miss a few salt mines. Be sure to watch out for the following:

Instant chocolate-flavored pudding. A half-cup contains 470 milligrams of sodium, more than the amount in two slices of bacon.

Cheese. Most varieties are high in sodium. This includes cottage cheese, which has 425 milligrams in a half-cup serving.

Pastries. A fruit Danish contains 333 milligrams of sodium; a cheese Danish, 319 milligrams. Scones and baking-powder biscuits also tend to be high in sodium.

Ketchup. One tablespoon has 156 milligrams of sodium.

When you go grocery shopping, be sure to look for foods that say "low-sodium" or "sodium-free" on their labels. And steer clear of anything extra-salty—especially canned vegetables and soups, lunchmeats, frozen dinners, and snack foods.

In addition, try to limit your use of table salt as much as possible. You can add flavor to your meals with liberal amounts of herbs and spices. (For some suggestions, see "Salt-Free Seasonings" on the opposite page.)

FOODS THAT FIGHT BACK

Rest assured, eating for a healthy blood pressure isn't all about "cutting back" or "giving up." If anything, you ought to be piling your plate with *more* of certain foods, especially the following. Their therapeutic properties can help erase points from your blood pressure reading. Research proves it!

Garlic. For benchmarks of heart health like blood pressure and cholesterol, "I don't know of any other natural substance that can duplicate the results of garlic," says Manfred Steiner, M.D., Ph.D., a hematologist now retired from East Carolina University in Greenville, North Carolina. For one study, Dr. Steiner had 41 volunteers supplement their diets with 7.2 grams of aged garlic extract—the equivalent of a clove of garlic— every day for 6 months. In that time, the participants' blood pressure dropped 5 to 6 percent, while their total and LDL cholesterol levels declined 7 to 8 percent. In addition, their blood platelets became less sticky, which reduced their risk of a heart attack or stroke.

According to Dr. Steiner, none of these improvements made a big difference by itself. But together, their effects were huge. To get similar results with medication, you'd need at least three different prescriptions. Dr. Steiner's findings bode well for people with slightly elevated blood pressure or cholesterol levels, and even for those with family histories of heart disease.

Garlic also appears to preserve the elasticity of arteries, which helps offset the stiffness and brittleness that can occur with lifelong exposure to dietary fat. In this condition, called arteriosclerosis, the arteries no longer can stretch to accommodate the blood pumping through them. So each heartbeat sends a wave of pressure throughout the body, leading to a form of high blood pressure that has been implicated in strokes and other cardiovascular problems.

In one study, German researchers compared 101 healthy adults who had taken garlic supplements—the equivalent of about half a clove of garlic every day for seven years—with people who hadn't. According to the researchers, the arteries of those in the garlic group were not nearly as stiff as the arteries of those in the control group.

Herb experts like James A. Duke, Ph.D., author of *The Green Pharmacy Anti-Aging Prescriptions,* recommend consuming about ½ ounce of garlic a week—or

---

PRESERVING GARLIC'S GOODNESS

So what's the best way to use garlic in your food? Garlic researcher John Milner, Ph.D., head of the nutrition department at Pennsylvania State University in University Park, offers these tips.

- Peel the clove before heating it. Otherwise, its various healing compounds won't form.
- Set aside the clove for 10 to 15 minutes after it's cut or crushed. This "breathing time" allows the all-important sulfurous compounds to form.

Be aware that garlic's healing compounds can linger in your body for several days. Since the herb thins the blood, you should limit yourself to two cloves a day if you're scheduled for surgery or you're taking anticoagulants.

---

about one whole clove a day—to help control blood pressure. If the herb is too pungent for your palate, even when mixed into food, you always can take it in supplement form. (For advice on choosing the right supplement, see page 81.)

Fish and other omega-3 sources. Eskimos thrive on one of the highest-fat diets in the world—heavy on roasted whale blubber, light on fruits, vegetables, and fiber. Plus, they're heavy smokers. You might expect them to be keeling over from heart attacks, one after the other. But they aren't. In fact, when researchers scoured ten years of health records from a hospital in Greenland that serves 2,000 people, they didn't find one death resulting from a heart attack.

The reason, scientists have since learned, is that the traditional Eskimo diet is rich in omega-3 fatty acids. On average, Eskimos consume 5 to 7 grams of eicosapentaenoic acid (EPA) and docosahexaenoic acid (DHA), two critical types of omega-3s, every day. But they don't get a lot of omega-6 fatty acids, found primarily in vegetable oils. That's good, because omega-6s can cancel out many of the good things omega-3s do.

"Heart disease, cancer, asthma, and autoimmune disorders occur less frequently in populations that eat more omega-3s and fewer omega-6s," confirms Artemis P. Simopoulos, M.D., president of the Center for Genetics, Nutrition, and Health in Washington, D.C., and author of *The Omega Diet.*

The best sources of omega-3s are fatty species of fish like salmon, tuna, and sardines. By eating up to three servings of fish per week *and* limiting your intake of saturated fat to about 25 percent of calories, you'll reduce your blood pressure even more than by only cutting back on total fat.

Not a fan of fish? You still can get omega-3s—albeit in smaller amounts—by eating walnuts or flaxseeds.

Calcium-rich foods. While most people know that getting enough calcium can help protect against osteoporosis, they don't realize that it also can help rein in high blood pressure. But a growing number of doctors are convinced that calcium has an anti-hypertensive effect, especially in those who are sensitive to sodium, says Michael Zemel, Ph.D., director of the Nutrition Institute at the University of Tennessee in Knoxville.

To maximize this effect, your best bet is to eat calcium-rich foods. "You get twice as big a reduction in blood pressure with dietary calcium as has ever been reported with calcium supplements," notes Robert P. Heaney, M.D., professor of medicine at the Osteoporosis Research Center at Creighton University in Omaha, Nebraska.

When 153 men and women followed a diet rich in fruits, vegetables, and low-fat dairy products, their blood pressure fell within days—more so than in people who followed a similar diet, only without the dairy. Dr. Heaney speculates that if everyone in the country ate the same sort of diet, with two to three servings of dairy a day, 27 percent fewer Americans would suffer strokes.

Bananas. The fruit that may be best known for its appeal to monkeys also happens to be a top-notch source of potassium, a mineral linked to lower blood pressure and a reduced risk of stroke.

When researchers at the Harvard School of Public Health tracked 43,738 men over eight years, they found that the men who had consumed the most potassium from foods had cut their risk of stroke by 38 percent. At least some of the mineral's apparent protective powers may come from its ability to lower blood pressure, notes Alberto Ascherio, M.D., Dr.P.H., assistant professor of nutrition and epidemiology at the Harvard School of Public Health.

Potassium also may help by discouraging LDL cholesterol from sticking to artery walls. This slows the formation of blockages that ultimately can shut off bloodflow to the brain, triggering a stroke.

You can get a hefty amount of potassium just by eating a banana a day. Other good sources of the mineral include baked potatoes, golden seedless raisins, and cantaloupe.

Celery. A handy vehicle for transporting peanut butter or cream cheese to your mouth, pale green, crunchy celery stalks make up for their lack of taste pizzazz with a plethora of phytonutrients. One of these is 3-n-butyl phthalide.

When researchers injected laboratory animals with a small amount of phthalide, the animals' blood pressure dropped 12 to 14 percent within a week. The nutrient works by relaxing muscles in the arterial walls, dilating the arteries and easing the pressure inside. Phthalide also reduces stress hormones in the blood, which typically elevate blood pressure by constricting arteries.

HOW TO WIN THE WEIGHT GAME

As mentioned at the start of the chapter, one of the "bonuses" of eating to lower your blood pressure is that you can lose those extra pounds. That's good, because being overweight is a major risk factor for high blood pressure and many of its complications.

Actually, most experts agree that the most effective approach to slimming down combines a healthy diet with regular physical activity. Keep in mind that to lose 1 pound, you need to eliminate 3,500 calories. The best way to do that is to eat a little less and exercise a little more every day. Aim to take off no more than ½ to 1 pound a week.

Whether you follow the menu plan in Chapter 8 or you decide to come up with your own, these tips can help keep your eating habits on track. (For advice on creating an exercise program, see Chapter 3.)

Keep a food diary for a week. People tend to underestimate how much they eat by 20 to 50 percent. That's a lot of extra calories! To get a better handle on your diet, try writing down everything you eat—both foods and portion sizes—every day for a week. Then look back over your notes. Chances are, you'll see distinct patterns of overeating, or perhaps unconscious nibbling. By figuring out when and why you overindulge, you can take steps to correct any behaviors that may interfere with your weight-loss efforts.

Bone up on portion sizes. Sure, you can count a heaping bowl of spaghetti as one serving. Just be prepared to do lots of exercise to burn off all those calories. Otherwise, you not only won't lose weight, you actually might end up *gaining*.

A SHOPPER'S GUIDE TO WHOLE GRAINS

Buying broccoli is easy, because you know it when you see it. Buying whole grains? You can't always believe your eyes. The hearty dark rye or seven-grain crackers that so convincingly appear to be whole grain may contain mostly refined white flour. To your body, that's the same as sugar.

To separate the (whole) wheat from the chaff, you need to read the ingredients list. What you see—or just as important, what you *don't* see—will determine whether you should buy a particular product or put it back on the shelf. Here's what to look for.

Wheat. The ingredients list should specify "whole wheat." If it doesn't, the product is made from refined wheat flour.

Oats. They're always whole oats, whether or not the label says so.

Rye. Look for the word "whole." In the United States, most rye and pumpernickel bread is made from refined wheat flour.

Corn. The ingredients list should specify "whole corn." Unfortunately, some products use whole corn but don't bother to mention it.

Rice. You should see the word "brown"; only brown varieties of rice are whole grain.

To make buying whole grains even easier, we've done a little shopping for you. Look for these products at your supermarket or health food store.

Bread
- Alvarado Street Bakery Sprouted Sourdough Bread
- Goya Corn Tortillas
- Matthew's Whole-Wheat English Muffins
- Mestemacher Three-Grain Bread
- Mestemacher Whole Rye Bread with Muesli
- Pepperidge Farm 100% Stone-Ground Whole Wheat Bread
- Thomas' Sahara 100% Whole-Wheat Pita Bread
- Wonder Stone-Ground 100% Whole-Wheat Bread

Cereal
- Arrowhead Mills Steel-Cut Oats
- General Mills Cheerios
- General Mills Wheat Chex
- Kellogg's Frosted Mini-Wheats
- Post Bran Flakes
- Post Raisin Bran
- Quaker Instant Oatmeal
- Quaker Old-Fashioned Oats
- Quaker Quick 1-Minute Oats

Crackers
- Ak-Mak Stone-Ground Sesame Crackers
- Kavli Hearty Thick Crispbread
- Ryvita Sesame Rye Crispbread
- Wasa Hearty Rye Original Crispbread
- Whole Foods Baked Woven Wheats

Pasta
- Annie's Whole-Wheat Shells and Cheddar
- DeCecco Whole-Wheat Linguine
- Fantastic Whole-Wheat Couscous
- Hodgson Mill Whole-Wheat Bow Tie
- Hodgson Mill Whole-Wheat Lasagna

Rice
- Fantastic Brown Basmati Rice
- Kraft Minute Instant Brown Rice
- Lundberg Family Farms Wehani Brown Rice
- Success 10-Minute Brown Rice
- Uncle Ben's Instant Brown Rice
- Wegmans Quick Cook Spanish Brown Rice

Snacks
- Bearitos Tortilla Chips
- New Morning Organic Cinnamon Grahams

The other option is to simply pay close attention to your portion sizes. Of course, you can't always measure the amount of food on your plate. But with practice, you can get a pretty good estimate just by eyeballing. These guidelines can help.

- Fresh or cooked vegetables: ½ cup, or about a rounded handful
- Raw or leafy vegetables: 1 cup, or the size of a baseball
- Fresh fruit: 1 medium piece, or the size of a baseball
- Cooked or canned fruit: ½ cup, or about a rounded handful
- Bread: 1 slice
- Ready-to-eat cereal: from ½ to 1¼ cups; check the nutrition label
- Cooked cereal: ½ cup, or about a rounded handful
- Cooked rice or pasta: ½ cup, or about a rounded handful
- Fish or meat: 3 ounces cooked (4 ounces raw), or the size of a deck of cards
- Dried beans: ½ cup cooked, or about a rounded handful
- Nuts: ⅓ cup, or about a level handful
- Cheese: 1½ ounces (2 ounces processed); 1 ounce is about the size of four dice

Eat from morning to night. If you plan to bypass breakfast to save on calories, your scheme will backfire. One study found that the metabolisms of people who skipped breakfast were about 5 percent lower than the metabolisms of people who ate at least three meals a day. A 5 percent increase in metabolism could lead to a 10-pound reduction in weight over the course of a year.

You can further bolster your weight-loss efforts by switching from the standard three square meals to smaller, more frequent meals spread over the course of a day. You're getting the same amount of food, but, because you're eating more often, you're less likely to feel hungry. In two separate studies, men who divvied up their breakfasts into "mini-meals" throughout the morning ate 27 percent less for lunch than men who had their breakfasts as a single meal.

Another good reason to avoid long stretches without food: After 4 hours, you'll experience a drop in blood sugar. You'll end up craving sweets, which rapidly convert to blood sugar, instead of healthier foods.

Triple your fiber intake. Your body will quickly absorb the calories from breakfast foods made with white flour and sugar, which means you'll feel hungry again soon after your meal. The calories from a bowl of bran cereal with no added sugar hang around longer, so you'll feel full longer. The same is true for other high-fiber foods.

Fiber also promotes weight loss by helping escort foods out of the body. Consider that your body absorbs about 4 fewer calories for every gram of fiber you eat, compared with a gram of simple carbohydrates.

Most people get about 13 grams of fiber a day. If you were to increase your intake to a little more than three times that amount, or 40 grams, you could block the absorption of 160 calories a day. Good sources of fiber include oatmeal, whole grains, beans, fruits, and vegetables.

Make water your beverage of choice. "A lot of people don't realize how many 'liquid calories' they consume," notes Ellen Albertson, R.D., cohost with husband Michael Albertson of the radio show *The Cooking Couple.* In one study, when people drank an extra 450 calories a day (as two gin and tonics or a cup of eggnog), they gained weight. But when they got those extra calories from food, they *lost* weight, because they ate less later in the day.

RUN AWAY FROM THIS VICE SQUAD

Just as certain foods can contribute to high blood pressure, so can certain substances. In particular, you may want to think twice about the following:

Alcohol. Drinking in moderation won't affect your blood pressure. In fact, it may be good for your heart and arteries, according to several studies. On the other hand, drinking in excess can cause long-term increases in blood pressure. In women, it also appears to raise the risk of breast cancer. The advice: If you don't drink, don't start. And if you do drink, limit yourself to 5 ounces of wine, 12 ounces of beer, or 1 ½ ounces of hard liquor a day.

Caffeine. Those who consume too much caffeine—in the form of coffee, tea, or cola—can experience rises in blood pressure of as much as 10 points. Your best bet is to switch to the decaf versions of your favorite beverages. If you absolutely need your caffeine, limit yourself to two servings of coffee, tea, or cola a day.

Nicotine. Every time you light up a cigarette, your blood pressure climbs—and it stays elevated for an hour or more afterward. So if you smoke, quit.

When you want to drink something, reach for a glass of water. You won't find a better thirst quencher. What's more, water has zero calories, it's filling, and it keeps your metabolism running efficiently.

CHAPTER FIVE

Stay a Step Ahead of Stress

Compared with other factors that can contribute to high blood pressure, stress doesn't get all that much attention from the national heart-health organizations. In fact, their view of the relationship between stress and high blood pressure is a decided departure from the conventional wisdom on the topic.

For example, experts at the National Heart, Lung, and Blood Institute say that while stress can cause a short-term rise in blood pressure, its long-term effects remain unclear. In addition, they contend that using stress-management techniques doesn't reduce the risk of high blood pressure.

So everyday tension and anxiety—the kind that crops up in the course of your normal routine—may not be as much of a factor in sustained high blood pressure as previously thought. That said, some people can develop high blood pressure because of more deep-seated, unresolved emotional issues.

"One-quarter to one-third of the hypertension cases in my practice are related to repressed or, so to speak, hidden emotions," says Samuel J. Mann, M.D., associate professor of clinical medicine at the Hypertension Center of New York Presbyterian Hospital/New York Weill Cornell Center in New York City and author of *Healing Hypertension.* "These are people who've experienced childhood traumas or who cope with emotional stress by ignoring it. They're the ones who are even-keeled, who never complain. And they actually are less likely than most to feel depressed."

People whose high blood pressure stems from unresolved emotional issues usually don't respond well to blood pressure medication. "Just shifting attention to those hidden emotions can rapidly lower blood pressure," Dr. Mann says. "Some people can heal themselves, while others benefit from consulting a psychotherapist."

THE HEART DISEASE CONNECTION

Even if stress doesn't play a major role in high blood pressure, it can have an enormous impact on other aspects of your health. For example, people burdened by chronic, uncontrolled stress are more likely to adopt unhealthy habits, such as overeating, smoking, and excessive drinking. They also are at greater risk for problems ranging from backache and bowel problems to headache and heart disease. In fact, cardiologist Alan Rozanski, M.D., director of nuclear cardiology and cardiac stress testing at St. Luke's–Roosevelt Hospital Center in New York City, describes stress as "a direct risk factor for heart disease, just like high blood pressure and cholesterol."

How can stress harm your heart? Essentially, by aggravating a process that already may be at work in your cardiovascular system.

Healthy arteries are as strong and flexible as rubber

bands, with inside surfaces as smooth as glass to facili-
tate bloodflow. But over time, they become hard and
narrow, and they develop scars. This scarring creates
ideal conditions for the accumulation of plaque—a
goopy mix of fat and cholesterol—on the artery walls,
which become as bumpy as a dirt road after an ice storm.
Eventually, the hard outer shell of the plaque may break
apart and block an artery, setting the stage for a blood
clot and possibly a heart attack or stroke.

The potential health implications of this process are
serious enough. Throw in chronic stress, and the situation gets even worse.

When you're feeling tense or anxious, your body re-
leases so-called stress hormones, such as adrenaline, no-
radrenaline, and cortisol. These hormones constrict
blood vessels and elevate heart rate and blood pressure.
Chronic stress can trigger repeated spikes in blood pressure, further damaging artery walls and increasing the
risk of heart disease.

Some studies suggest that stress also has an effect on
cholesterol. In particular, both short-term and long-term
stress can raise LDL cholesterol, the bad kind, says
Catherine M. Stoney, Ph.D., professor of psychology at
Ohio State University in Columbus. Dr. Stoney has been
examining the relationship between psychological stress
and cholesterol for more than a decade. As early as the
1950s, studies showed that race-car drivers had higher
cholesterol levels after competition. More recently, Dr.
Stoney found that airline pilots studying for their recer-
tification exam had higher cholesterol levels prior to the
test.

Dr. Stoney also found that stress elevates levels of
homocysteine, an amino acid that appears to cause thick-
ening and scarring of the artery linings. In one study
involving 34 healthy women between ages 40 and 63,

Dr. Stoney documented increases in homocysteine when the women gave a speech before a camera or subtracted backward by 13—both researchers' techniques for creating stress. Afterward, levels of the amino acid dropped back to normal.

The bottom line: Until scientists learn more about the precise role of stress in high blood pressure, you should practice good stress management just for the sake of lowering your overall risk of heart disease. With that in mind, let's explore some effective strategies for coping with two common sources of stress: career and family.

SURVIVING TODAY'S WORKPLACE

Nearly half of all American workers experience symptoms of burnout, a disabling reaction to stress on the job, says Naomi Swanson, Ph.D., chief of the work organization and stress research section of the National Institute for Occupational Safety and Health in Cincinnati. And stress on the job is more rampant than ever, as companies everywhere downsize, outsource, and restructure, leaving their employees feeling frustrated, alienated, and insecure.

For proof, consider these findings from the American Institute of Stress in Yonkers, New York.

- On an average workday, an estimated 1 million workers are absent because of stress-related complaints.
- Of the 550 million workdays lost to absenteeism each year, stress is thought to be responsible for more than half.
- A 3-year study conducted by a large corporation found that 60 percent of employee absences were due to psychological problems such as stress.

In general, stress occurs when our jobs fail to meet our expectations. Most of us try to fix the mismatch by changing our responses to stress-provoking situations. That's a good start. But research has shown that to avoid burnout, we also need to take steps to alleviate stress at the source: the job itself. These tips can help.

Take the lead. You can't turn around your workplace all by yourself. But you can jump-start the process by taking on a leadership role. Your first step is to pinpoint the ways in which your job creates stress, Dr. Swanson advises.

Research has shown that different occupations tend to generate different stressors. Among nurses, for example, the main issue is conflict with colleagues. Among clerical workers, it's lack of control. Incidentally, research also has shown that employees who feel lots of stress but have little control over their jobs are at greater risk for developing high blood pressure and experiencing a heart attack.

Reach out to coworkers. "To make an impact, you'll need to approach change as a group project," explains Christina Maslach, Ph.D., professor of psychology at the University of California, Berkeley. Arrange a meeting with coworkers to share concerns, but try not to let it turn into a gripe session. Instead, use the time to identify one problem that everyone wants to address first. Usually, it's the one with the highest potential for burnout. Then discuss realistic, concrete solutions.

Improve your own marketability. Network within your company, enroll in a class at your local community college, or hire a tutor to improve your skills. Any of these strategies can increase your sense of control over your situation. They also foster the necessary confidence to tackle new challenges and handle the unexpected.

Punch out earlier. In many segments of the American workforce, the norm is to hang around the office until the cleaning staff comes in. But the latest research suggests that grueling hours are no longer a prerequisite for career success. According to one study, more than one-third of employees who choose to work reduced hours receive promotions anyway. What's more, 70 percent of supervisors supported employees who wanted to work fewer hours.

Learn to detach. In some professions, like nursing and social work, the risk of burnout runs especially high. That's when you need to develop detached concern, according to Beverly Potter, Ph.D., a psychologist in Berkeley, California, and author of *Overcoming Job Burnout.* In other words, you focus on your efforts and let go of the results.

"When Mother Teresa was asked how she could stand to work with sick and dying children, she is reported to have said, 'I love them while they are here,' " Dr. Potter says. "Her love was the concern, and the 'while they are here' was her detachment."

NAVIGATING MARITAL MINEFIELDS

It ain't about the dishes.

If you dig deep enough, you'll find that all those minor marital squabbles over seemingly insignificant transgressions have their roots in the common ground of basic human needs. "From the day we're born, we try to satisfy our own needs," explains Allen Fay, M.D., a psychiatrist in New York City and author of *Making It as a Couple.*

That's why all married couples seem to bicker about the same issues: sex, money, children, extended family, outside friendships and other relationships, household chores, work, spirituality, and health. The trick is not to

TRAVEL THERAPY

If you haven't taken a vacation lately, you had better start making plans—and soon. New research shows that an annual getaway literally could save your life.

Every year for five years, 12,000 men at high risk for heart disease completed questionnaires that asked, among other things, whether they had gone on vacation in the previous twelve months. The more frequently the men answered yes, the less likely they were to die of any cause—and particularly of heart disease—in the subsequent nine years.

A vacation may safeguard your health simply because it's downtime, when you can destress for days on end, speculates lead researcher Brooks Gump, Ph.D., assistant professor of psychology at the State University of New York at Oswego. Studies have proven that stress can raise the risk of a range of illnesses, including heart disease.

To get the most from your time off, follow this advice.

Make it a regular event. The questionnaire in the study didn't ask how often the men went on vacation. In general, once a year is a good benchmark, Dr. Gump says. A week or more may be ideal, but even a long weekend can help.

Leave behind the laptop. Especially if you're under stress, you shouldn't take your computer—or any work, for that matter—on your trip, Dr. Gump says. It defeats the purpose of getting away. For the same reason, resist the urge to check in with the office, and don't leave a number where you can be reached.

Take your buddies. Vacations may be beneficial because they provide an opportunity to spend quality time with family and friends. Studies have found that social support and strong interpersonal relationships can reduce the risk of heart disease and other health problems, Dr. Gump notes.

Or enjoy solitude. If spending a week with extended family or certain other folks in your social sphere only adds to your tension and anxiety, then by all means leave home without them.

Get away every day. If you just can't escape for a week

or even a long weekend, schedule a 15-minute "micro-vacation" every day. "Put a sign on your office door that says you'll be back in 15 minutes," Dr. Gump suggests. "Then close the door, disconnect your phone, turn off your e-mail, and relax." Practice deep breathing, read a novel, listen to music—or simply do nothing at all.

let these disagreements mushroom to the point where they erode the marriage itself. The following strategies can help resolve conflicts, relieve stress, and restore harmony between you and your spouse.

Use fuzzy math. "A marriage is not a 50/50 proposition," Dr. Fay notes. "It's a 60/60 proposition. Each person has to do a little more than what he or she thinks is a fair share." And don't keep score. It will only eat away at your happiness.

Don't look back. The past is valuable for only two things: recalling pleasant experiences and learning from mistakes. "If a deed was so bad that you feel you must end your relationship because of it, by all means do so," Dr. Fay says. "But if you choose to stay with your partner, tell yourself to forget it, and don't hassle him or her about it." Harboring resentment about the past only undermines the promise of the present and future.

Count to 10. During a discussion with your spouse, especially a heated one, wait 10 seconds before responding. "The 10-second rule slows our minds a little bit, putting a pause into our interactions with others," says Albert Couch, founding partner of Signal Tree Resolutions mediation center in Akron, Ohio, and mediator of more than 1,200 family and organization negotiations. "If I wait before I respond, I'll be listening, not thinking about what I'm going to say. I have 10 seconds to do that."

FOR YOUR HEART'S SAKE, FORGIVE

Forgiveness can do more than mend strained relationships. One new study has shown that it can immediately and dramatically improve physical health, too.

For the study, researchers at Hope College in Holland, Michigan, asked 71 people to mentally relive hurtful memories, with two different endings: one in which they held a grudge, the other in which they forgave the offending parties. The study participants thought about their friends, romantic partners, parents, and siblings. Common offenses included betrayal of trust, rejection, lies, and insults.

During the study, the researchers tracked the participants' heart rates, blood pressure levels, and perspiration. They also probed their subjects' emotions.

The researchers determined that heart rates and blood pressure levels were 2½ times lower when the study volunteers forgave compared with when they held a grudge. Holding a grudge also made the participants sweat, a sign their nervous systems were on high alert. Forgiveness left them feeling calm and in control. "They were much more negative, angry, and sad when they didn't forgive than when they did," notes Charlotte van Oyen Witvliet, Ph.D., assistant professor of psychology at Hope College.

What's the significance of these findings? "We know that sustained anger and hostility are risk factors for heart disease," Dr. Witvliet says. "Forgiveness may be a powerful antidote. People can experience health benefits when they become forgiving, just as they experience health risks when they harbor anger and hostility."

Fake it. If you can't seem to resolve a particular issue, call a 1-week truce. "Behavior can precede change," Dr. Fay notes. Some couples need no more than a few style changes to bring about marked and lasting improvement in their relationships. So pretend you've solved the problem—and add a compliment and a couple of long hugs every day. How angry will you feel then?

WHAT ABOUT THE KIDS?

It's ironic, really. Many couples spend weeks attending childbirth classes to prepare for the first day of a child's life. But they get little, if any, training to prepare for the subsequent 18 years!

Children, as much as we love them, can bring very real stress into our lives. Mastering our relationships with them is all the more difficult because it isn't like riding a bike. Parenting doesn't teach skills that we can retain and use throughout life. Sure, we think we're getting the parenting stuff down pat. But our children keep growing up, and the rules keep changing.

We need to learn how to handle the challenges if we want to thrive as parents and do right by our kids. While no one solution fits every situation, these tips can help maintain a sense of calm and control on the home front.

First and foremost, pay attention. Scheduling "quality time" isn't enough. If you want your child to open up to you, then you need to listen to him. It shows respect for his feelings, and it bolsters his self-esteem.

And when your child talks, don't interrupt—even if he slips in a curse word or mentions engaging in an activity that you don't approve of. For the moment, your job is to listen, not cast judgment. If you want to express another point of view, do so with respect, not condescension.

Avoid lecturing. Parents and teens can have a particularly difficult time communicating with one another. You can help ease conversations with your teenager by making sure that your comments are at least 50 percent positive or neutral, suggests Vickie Beck, a nurse/psychotherapist and consultant to Mercy Hospital in Baltimore. In other words, no more than half of your comments should focus on potentially divisive issues like setting limits or following rules.

Reward responsibility. Your children may balk at having to earn certain privileges. But if you come up with a set of ground rules and stick with them, you'll earn your kids' respect, says Katherine Kersey, Ph.D., professor of education and chairperson of the department of child studies at Old Dominion University in Norfolk, Virginia.

Dr. Kersey recalls that when her children were younger, they had to make their beds before they could play outside. Two of her kids made their beds every morning, but the third waited until after school. And if it was raining, he decided that he didn't need to make his bed, because he couldn't play outside anyway. He may have been flexing his independence, but he knew the rule, and he abided by it.

Get help if you need it. A stressed-out parent has every right to seek out advice and support from others, says Aletha Solter, Ph.D., a developmental psychologist who runs the Aware Parenting Institute in Goleta, California. She recommends consulting people who know and love you and your child, such as parents, grandparents, siblings, and other relatives. You also might enlist the assistance of a close friend, a member of the clergy, a professional therapist, your child's guidance counselor, a support group, or a community social services agency. Even a good book on child behavior or parenting can be an indispensable resource for navigating particularly treacherous parental terrain.

Forgo the guilt. Every new generation of parents seems determined to provide their children with the sorts of things that they didn't have when they were growing up. Just remember that in the long run, good parenting skills—spending time with your kids, listening to them, encouraging them—are much more valuable than the size of your bank account.

THE HEALING POWER OF MEDITATION

Even in the midst of a stressful situation, you can take steps to defuse your body's stress response. And it doesn't involve quitting your job, leaving your spouse, or sending your kids to boarding school. Instead, just meditate. In only a few minutes a day, it can chase away cares and concerns better than soaking in a bath full of bubbles.

The health benefits of meditation first began appearing in the medical literature more than twenty-five years ago. Most notably, meditation relaxes blood vessels, which can help rein in high blood pressure. One particular study found that learning to relieve stress through meditation could reduce the risk of atherosclerosis and, with it, the risk of heart attack and stroke.

You can achieve a meditative state—which emphasizes "being" rather than "doing"—using a number of different techniques. Among the more popular are the following:

Transcendental meditation. Also known as TM, this form of meditation can produce a significant reduction in blood pressure in as little as three months. Some studies involving African-Americans—who are at especially high risk for high blood pressure—have shown declines of as much as 11 points systolic (the top number in a blood pressure reading) and 6 points diastolic (the bottom number).

"Transcendental meditation works by promoting a

state of 'restful alertness' in mind and body," explains Charles Alexander, Ph.D., professor of psychology and codirector of the Center for Health and Aging Studies at the Maharishi University of Management in Fairfield, Iowa. "This state is beneficial to the physiological systems affected by the wear and tear of stress."

During a TM session, you sit comfortably, close your eyes, and concentrate on a mantra, a meaningless sound or a word or phrase. This gently shifts your attention away from external distractions and toward your innermost thoughts, Dr. Alexander explains. Eventually, your mind transcends even the internal thinking process and becomes completely silent.

Research has shown that when practiced for 15 to 20 minutes twice a day, TM can produce a spectrum of health benefits, including a reduction in the symptoms of heart disease. You can learn more about TM by contacting the Maharishi Vedic university, college, school, or center closest to your hometown. Call (888) 532-7686, or visit www.maharishi.org and click on "MVU Locations."

Mindfulness meditation. Also known as nonconcentrative meditation, mindfulness meditation has its roots in Buddhist traditions. Unlike TM, it does not necessarily lead to a deeply relaxed state. Instead, it promotes greater self-awareness by tuning in to the body's moment-to-moment changes. And it's easy to practice on your own.

First, you need to find a sitting position that will be comfortable for 10 to 15 minutes. Then take several deep breaths, slowly inhaling and exhaling through your nose. But avoid controlling your breathing; it should follow a natural rhythm. Next, start counting—1 when you inhale, 2 when you exhale, 3 when you inhale, and so on until you reach 10. Don't get frustrated if you lose count. Just return to 1 and start again.

Once you reach a point where you no longer lose count (which may take a month or two of practice), you can simplify your meditation by saying "in" when you inhale and "out" when you exhale. You also can expand your focus to include other sensory perceptions—sights, smells, temperature, and the like.

Progressive relaxation. In this form of meditation, you alternately contract and release each major muscle group, with the goal of completely relaxing your entire body. It's especially helpful if you're having trouble sleeping at night.

To begin, lie down or sit in a dark, quiet room. Tense a muscle group—for example, the one in your right arm. Hold for 15 seconds, then release, exhaling as you do. After a brief rest, move on to another muscle group, working your way through every muscle in your body.

Guided imagery. As its name suggests, this technique involves the use of mental images to bring about relaxation. Need a vacation? Thanks to guided imagery, you can get away without ever leaving home. Just settle into a comfortable position and picture yourself in your favorite destination—the beach, for example. Feel the soft sand between your toes, the warm sun on your face, the cool ocean spray in your hair. The more detailed your image is, the more convinced your body will be that you actually are there.

As for how long your mini-vacation should last, that's really up to you. 30 to 60 minutes is ideal, but if you don't have that much time, even 5 to 10 minutes can do the trick. Again, it depends how detailed your image is.

PART III

Remedies That Pack a Punch

CHAPTER SIX

The Best of the Blood Pressure Drugs

In many cases, lifestyle strategies alone can reduce blood pressure to an acceptable level. But what if your reading remains stubbornly high, despite your committed efforts to eat healthfully, exercise regularly, and destress as much as possible? Under the circumstances, you may need to add medication to your blood pressure–management plan.

These days, your doctor can choose from all kinds of prescription blood pressure drugs—each with a distinct action in the body, most (if not all) with side effects. You could end up trying several different drugs to find the one that best suits your particular situation.

Generally, once you start taking medication, you must stay on it for the rest of your life, even after you rein in your blood pressure. If you were to stop treatment, your reading probably would climb right back to an unhealthy level. The good news is that you may be able to reduce your dosage—with your doctor's approval and supervision—once your blood pressure stays in the normal range (below 120/80) for at least a year.

With all this in mind, let's take a closer look at the

HOW ABOUT AN ASPIRIN NIGHTCAP?

If you're using aspirin to help control your blood pressure, be aware that what time you take it can have a noticeable effect on how well it works. In a study at the University Clinical Hospital of Santiago de Compostela in Spain, patients with high blood pressure who took their aspirin before going to bed saw much greater reductions in their readings than patients who took it in the morning or at other times of day.

Aspirin's benefits peak within 4 to 6 hours—just in time to counteract the early-morning rise in proteins that constricts blood vessels and increases blood pressure. A low-dose aspirin (about 100 milligrams) is enough to help reduce a mildly elevated reading.

---

most popular categories of blood pressure drugs—how they work, what generic and brand names they go by, and what side effects they may cause. While you still need a doctor's prescription for your medication, you can use the information to comparison shop and narrow your choices. (If you're already taking medication, you may want to consider switching, based on what you read here.)

Diuretics. The drugs in this category lower blood pressure by flushing sodium and water from the body, which reduces the amount of sodium in the blood. Typically, doctors prescribe diuretics in combination with other blood pressure medications.

Government-sponsored research reported in the *Journal of the American Medical Association* concluded that so-called thiazide-type diuretics should be the first choice among all drugs in treating high blood pressure. The reason: They're more effective and less expensive than their newer brethren.

HRT AND THE FEMALE HEART

For years the medical community has been engaged in a heated debate about the use of hormone replacement therapy (HRT) for hot flashes, insomnia, mood swings, and other common menopausal discomforts. The controversy reached its boiling point in July 2002, when researchers abruptly terminated a huge federal study investigating the long-term safety of hormone replacement. The reason for the sudden stop: The women in the study who took combination HRT (estrogen plus progestin) showed an increased risk of heart disease, stroke, and blood clots, as well as invasive breast cancer.

Despite these findings, many top experts believe that the majority of women can safely use combination HRT for 2 to 3 years to relieve menopausal discomforts. But this general guideline does have its exceptions. In particular, if you have any risk factors for heart disease, stroke, or blood clots, you are not a candidate for hormone replacement. According to the federal study, the risk for all three conditions climbed highest in the first two years of HRT.

You also should consider other treatment options for your menopausal discomforts if you have a personal history of breast cancer or any risk factors for the disease. If you decide to try combination HRT, keep it short-term.

Incidentally, the combination HRT in the federal study consisted of 0.625 milligram of conjugated equine estrogens (Premarin) plus 2.5 milligrams of medroxyprogesterone acetate (Provera). Using a different combination or different dosages could affect the associated disease risk.

Ultimately, you and your doctor need to weigh the pros and cons of HRT in light of your particular health situation before you decide whether or not to try it. If you're already using HRT and you want to quit, don't do it abruptly. Work with your doctor to come up with a plan for tapering off.

Diuretics can deplete the body's potassium supply, causing fatigue, weakness, and leg cramps. To compensate for this side effect, pharmaceutical companies developed potassium-sparing diuretics such as amiloride (Midamor), triamterene (Dyrenium), and spironolactone (Aldactone). As their name suggests, these drugs don't affect the body's potassium levels.

Another type of potassium-sparing diuretic contains two different diuretic agents. The drugs in this category include Aldactazide, Dyazide, Moduretic, and Maxzide.

The most common side effects of the potassium-sparing diuretics are stomach upset, diarrhea, nausea, and vomiting. With these drugs, you also need to watch for signs of a sodium shortfall—most notably drowsiness, mouth dryness, and increased thirst.

Beta-blockers. The name *beta-blockers* comes from the much more imposing *beta-adrenergic blocking agents*. These drugs work by minimizing nerve impulses to the heart and blood vessels, which reduces the force and frequency of the heartbeat. As a result, your blood pressure drops, since your heart doesn't need to work as hard.

Beta-blockers are sold under a number of generic and brand names. They include atenolol (Tenormin), metoprolol (Lopressor), and timolol (Blocadren).

Among the side effects associated with beta-blockers are fatigue, insomnia, depression, and cold hands and feet. The drugs also can trigger asthma symptoms and, in people with diabetes, may interfere with insulin therapy.

ACE inhibitors. The "ACE" in ACE inhibitors stands for angiotensin-converting enzyme. These drugs block the formation of angiotensin II, a hormone that plays a role in narrowing blood vessels. Instead, the blood vessels relax, so your blood pressure drops.

BEFORE YOU POP THAT PILL . . .

Whenever your doctor hands over a prescription—whether for high blood pressure or another condition—take a moment to ask some basic questions about it. They won't take long, and they can help ensure that you're using your medication safely and effectively.

- What are the brand and generic names of the medication?
- What is the correct dosage?
- When should I take it?
- How should I take it—with food or on an empty stomach?
- What are the side effects? What should I do if I notice any of them?
- Could this medication interact with other drugs I'm taking?
- Could it interact with any foods or herbal or nutritional supplements?
- Should I avoid alcohol while on the medication?
- What if I miss a dose?

Among the drugs in this category are enalapril (Vasotec), quinapril (Accupril), and benazepril (Lotensin). Their side effects range from skin rash and chronic coughing to an impaired sense of taste and, in rare cases, kidney damage.

Angiotensin II receptor antagonists. One of the newer categories of blood pressure drugs, the angiotensin II receptor antagonists disrupt the action of angiotensin II. Though they work a bit differently than the ACE inhibitors, the outcome is the same: Blood vessels relax, and blood pressure drops.

The drugs valsartan (Diovan), candesartan (Atacand), and irbesartan (Avapro) all fall into the category of angiotensin II receptor antagonists. So far, their most common side effect appears to be occasional dizziness.

Calcium channel blockers. As their name implies, these drugs prevent calcium from entering the muscle cells in your heart and blood vessels. This action allows the blood vessels to relax.

The calcium channel blockers go by a number of names, such as amlodipine (Norvasc), diltiazem (Cardizem CD), and felodipine (Plendil). Their known side effects include ankle swelling, constipation, headache, and heart palpitations.

Alpha-blockers. Drugs in this category—such as doxazosin (Cardura) and terazosin (Hytrin)—interfere with the transmission of nerve impulses to blood vessels. This relaxes the blood vessels and improves bloodflow.

Based on a clinical study, experts at the National Heart, Lung, and Blood Institute advise against using alpha-blockers as a first-line treatment in cases of high blood pressure with no complications. And if you experience any dizziness or increase in heart rate while taking one of these drugs, be sure to report it to your doctor.

Alpha-beta blockers. These drugs work much like the alpha-blockers, except they also slow the heartbeat, like the beta-blockers. With the heart pumping less blood through the blood vessels, blood pressure declines.

Both carvedilol (Coreg) and labetalol (Normodyne) are alpha-beta blockers. Taking these drugs can cause blood pressure to drop if you stand up too quickly, resulting in dizziness or loss of balance.

Nervous system inhibitors. By regulating nerve impulses, the nervous system inhibitors—such as guanadrel (Hylorel), guanethidine (Ismelin), and reserpine (Serpasil)—help relax and dilate blood vessels. This improves bloodflow and reduces blood pressure.

As with the alpha-beta blockers, the nervous system inhibitors can cause dizziness or weakness if you stand

MEDICATION REMINDERS

In general, blood pressure medications work best when they're taken on a regular schedule—at about the same time of day every day. To avoid missing a dose, try one or more of these memory devices from the National Institutes of Health.

- Link your medication to another daily activity, like showering or brushing your teeth. If you must take your pill with food, pair it with the same meal every day.
- Post reminder notes in obvious places—on the refrigerator, by the phone, on the medicine cabinet, or even on the bathroom mirror.
- Use a calendar or chart to track your medication. Keep it someplace handy so that you can mark when you've taken your pills for the day. If you're on multiple medications, choose a different color pen for each one. Also note when you're due for your next refill.
- Buy one of those special pillboxes that divvy your medication into daily doses. Most drugstores and many discount department stores sell them.
- If you have voicemail service on your telephone, record a reminder message about your medication. The service will automatically call at the designated time each day.
- Establish a buddy system with a family member or friend who also takes medication. Make plans to call each other at designated times each day.
- If you spend a lot of time on your computer, enter your medication schedule as appointments on your electronic calendar. Or sign up for a free service that will send reminder e-mails on a daily basis.

up too quickly. Other known side effects include diarrhea and, for reserpine, nasal congestion and heartburn.

Vasodilators. Often doctors prescribe vasodilators in combination with other blood pressure medications. The vasodilators work by relaxing the muscle in the blood vessel walls, which leads to a decline in blood pressure.

Among the drugs in this category is hydralazine (Apresoline), which can trigger heart palpitations, headaches, and joint pain. Typically, these side effects subside within a few weeks of beginning treatment.

CHAPTER SEVEN

The Natural Route to Healthy Blood Pressure

For the most serious cases of high blood pressure, when readings hover at or above 140/90, medication may be the fastest route to control the condition and head off potentially life-threatening complications. But what if you're dealing with a relatively mild case—say, at the lower end of the prehypertensive range (120/80 to 139/89)? You may want to explore another treatment option: natural medicine.

Certain herbs and nutritional supplements can lower blood pressure as effectively as prescription pharmaceuticals, especially in combination with the sorts of lifestyle strategies discussed in Part II. Even better, natural remedies tend to have fewer side effects than drugs.

On the other hand, they do work more slowly than conventional medications. And they can cause troublesome interactions, inhibiting or intensifying the actions of certain drugs. For these reasons, you should consult a physician who's knowledgeable about herbs and nutritional supplements before adding them to your self-care regimen.

Among the natural remedies said to lower blood pressure, these eleven have particularly potent therapeutic power.

Hawthorn. The leaves, berries, and flowers of the hawthorn tree get a standing ovation for their cardiovascular health benefits. Do those benefits include lowering blood pressure? You bet.

"Hawthorn is one of the most commonly recommended herbs for hypertension," says Ian Bier, N.D., Ph.D., a naturopathic physician in Portsmouth, New Hampshire. "It's very powerful, yet very gentle. While it needs time, it does work." In fact, hawthorn works much like conventional blood pressure medications, only without the side effects.

To treat high blood pressure, look for hawthorn capsules that are standardized to a flavonoid (a natural plant nutrient) called vitexin, advises Robert Rountree, M.D., a holistic physician at the Helios Health Center in Boulder, Colorado. Take two 500-milligram capsules three times a day to start. As your blood pressure drops, reduce your dosage to one capsule three times a day, then to one capsule twice a day.

You can buy hawthorn tincture—made by soaking the herb's leaves in alcohol or glycerin to extract their medicinal compounds—but it isn't as potent as the capsules, Dr. Rountree says. If you prefer the tincture, take 1 teaspoon three times a day, mixed into some water. As with the capsules, you can taper your dosage as your blood pressure drops—first to ½ teaspoon of tincture three times a day, then to ½ teaspoon twice a day.

Note: Be sure to check your blood pressure at least once every two weeks while you're taking hawthorn. As a general rule, people with high blood pressure or other cardiovascular conditions should limit their use of hawthorn to a few weeks, unless they're under medical supervision.

Garlic. "Garlic is a good example of an herb that is common in the diet and helpful as a botanical medicine," says George Milowe, M.D., a holistic physician in Saratoga Springs, New York. "Studies have proven that it lowers blood pressure."

For people who have healthy blood pressure and want to keep it that way, Dr. Rountree recommends eating a clove of garlic—preferably raw—every day, either alone or as an ingredient in another dish. If you have high blood pressure, though, you want your garlic a bit more potent. You can get that potency by taking four to six 600-milligram garlic capsules or tablets every day, in divided doses.

This may seem like a simple enough prescription. But it can get confusing, primarily because different manufacturers use different processing methods to produce their garlic supplements. And those processing methods influence the supplements' potency.

Your best bet is to choose a garlic product that's standardized to allicin. Actually, you'll measure your dosage in "allicin potential," because certain compounds in garlic convert to allicin in the body. Dr. Rountree recommends getting the equivalent of 8,000 micrograms of allicin potential every day.

You probably will need to continue therapy for at least a month before you see results. Fortunately, garlic is safe enough that it can be taken indefinitely—though, because it thins the blood, it should be used with caution by anyone who's on prescription anticoagulants or who's scheduled for surgery. Be sure to talk with your doctor.

To learn more about the beneficial relationship between garlic and blood pressure, see page 43.

Coenzyme Q_{10}. Its alternative name, ubiquinone, alludes to the fact that coenzyme Q_{10} is ubiquitous—that is, it's everywhere in the body. Basically, it serves as a catalyst for the cellular reactions that support the production of ATP, the energy source for cells. ATP juices up the heart muscle cells, which pump with greater efficiency and less effort. This, in turn, helps lower blood pressure.

The recommended dosage for coenzyme Q_{10} is 100 milligrams a day. (Dosages of more than 120 milligrams a day require medical supervision, especially if taken for more than 20 days.) Potential side effects include heartburn, nausea, and stomachache—all of which can be avoided simply by taking supplements with meals. In rare instances, coenzyme Q_{10} can interfere with the blood thinner warfarin (Coumadin), reducing the effectiveness of the drug.

Onion. It may not be quite as pungent as its cousin, garlic. But onion does have similar benefits for lowering blood pressure, according to herb expert James A. Duke, Ph.D., author of *The Green Pharmacy Anti-Aging Prescriptions.*

In studies, taking 2 to 3 tablespoons of onion oil a day produced significant improvement in the blood pressure readings of two-thirds of people with moderately high blood pressure, Dr. Duke says. Another option is to lightly cook either 2 ounces of fresh onion or 1 ounce of dried onion, then eat it "as is" or mix it into food.

Fish oil. Scientists have yet to figure out exactly how fish oil lowers blood pressure and protects against heart disease. But many suspect it has something to do with fish oil's ability to thin the blood, which reduces the risk of clots. Fish oil also may counteract inflammation and help relax arteries.

You can get your fish oil straight from the source: fatty fish like salmon, tuna, and sardines. But if you're not crazy about "fin food," you have another option:

supplements. Aim for about 720 milligrams of eicosa-pentaenoic acid (EPA) and 480 milligrams of docosah-exaenoic acid (DHA)—both omega-3 fatty acids—every day. You may need to take several capsules a day to get this amount; be sure to read the product label for the proper dosage.

Note: Experts advise against fish-oil supplements for people with seriously high blood pressure, bleeding disorders, or allergies to fish. The supplements also are not appropriate for people who take anticoagulants (blood thinners) or aspirin on a regular basis.

For more information about the role of fish and fish oil in controlling blood pressure, see page 45.

Dill. According to Dr. Duke, dill seeds contain an oil that acts as a diuretic. As you may recall from Chapter 6, diuretics help eliminate fluid from the body, reducing blood volume and lowering blood pressure.

You can use fresh or dried dill straight from your spice rack, Dr. Duke says. Or brew a dill tea: Steep 1 to 3 teaspoons of crushed dill seed in a cup of freshly boiled water for 10 minutes, then strain out the seed and let cool before drinking. Be aware that dill contains a substantial amount of sodium. You probably should avoid it if you're on a low-sodium diet.

Mushrooms. Natural-minded physicians count on an all-star lineup of medicinal mushrooms to treat and prevent a whole host of ailments. For high blood pressure, the mushroom of choice is reishi. "I frequently recommend reishi for blood pressure, as both a tonic [a preventive] and a medicinal," Dr. Rountree says. "It is very safe, and it has all kinds of other benefits, too."

You can buy reishi capsules in health food stores and by mail order. Dr. Rountree suggests finding a product with a strong enough concentration that you get 2,000 to 4,000 milligrams a day without swallowing too many capsules. You can continue taking reishi indefinitely.

Motherwort. Practitioners of Traditional Chinese Medicine depend on the flowering herb motherwort to rein in high blood pressure. "It directly lowers blood pressure, and it has a calming effect," Dr. Rountree says.

Most health food stores sell motherwort in tincture form. According to Dr. Rountree, the typical dosage is 2 or 3 dropperfuls a day. (The tincture comes with a dropper attached to the lid.) You can take it straight or mix it into a glass of water.

Ginkgo. It may be best known as a "brain herb." But ginkgo has cardiovascular benefits, too. "It dilates the peripheral blood vessels, and any substance that does that will automatically lower blood pressure by giving the blood more room to move through," Dr. Bier says. "I would definitely throw ginkgo into a formula with hawthorn."

You can make your own formula from tinctures, using twice as much hawthorn as ginkgo. The simplest recipe is to buy a 1-ounce bottle of ginkgo and a 2-ounce bottle of hawthorn and combine the two. Take a teaspoon of the formula three times a day, mixed with a little water.

While ginkgo rarely causes side effects, it can inhibit the blood's ability to clot. For this reason, it is not recommended for people who are taking a blood-thinning medication such as warfarin (Coumadin) or a regular therapeutic dose of aspirin.

Evening primrose. The oil from evening primrose seeds contains gamma-linolenic acid, an essential fatty acid that helps lower blood pressure, Dr. Duke says. You can buy capsules containing the oil. Follow the label instructions for proper dosage.

Devil's claw. In studies involving laboratory animals, the herb devil's claw has had a beneficial effect on blood pressure, Dr. Duke notes. He suggests making a tea by steeping 1 to 2 teaspoons of the herb in a cup of freshly boiled water. Then strain out the herb and drink up— one or two cups a day.

If you have ulcers, you should steer clear of devil's claw, which can aggravate the condition. Gallstones also warrant extra caution; in that case, you'll want to check with your doctor before taking the herb.

PART IV

**The Outsmart High Blood Pressure
Eating Plan**

CHAPTER EIGHT

Ditch Points with the DASH Diet

The experts at the National Heart, Lung, and Blood Institute have developed a week's worth of menu plans that adhere to the basic guidelines of the DASH diet. As you may recall from Chapter 4, DASH stands for Dietary Approaches to Stop Hypertension. Research has proven the diet to be extraordinarily effective in reducing elevated blood pressure, often within a matter of weeks.

The menus in the plan supply approximately 2,000 calories a day, give or take a few. If you need to consume fewer than that—because you're trying to lose weight, for example—simply reduce your serving sizes. Have room for a few more calories? Then increase your serving sizes.

As for sodium, which can elevate blood pressure even in people with normal readings, the menus supply roughly 2,400 milligrams a day. You can reduce this amount to about 1,500 milligrams by making the substitutions and adjustments that appear in *italic*.

Day 1
Breakfast
⅔ cup bran cereal or *⅔ cup shredded wheat cereal*
1 slice whole wheat bread with 2 teaspoons jelly
1 medium banana
1 cup no-sugar-added, fat-free fruit yogurt
1 cup fat-free milk

Lunch
Chicken salad sandwich made with ¾ cup Chicken Salad, *remove the salt from the recipe* (see page 128); 1 tablespoon Dijon mustard or *1 tablespoon regular mustard*; and 2 slices whole wheat bread
Salad made with ½ cup fresh cucumber slices, ½ cup tomato wedges, and 2 tablespoons fat-free ranch dressing or *2 tablespoons yogurt dressing*
½ cup fruit cocktail, juice pack

Dinner
3 ounces eye of round beef with 2 tablespoons low-fat beef gravy or *2 tablespoons unsalted, low-fat beef gravy*
1 small baked potato topped with 2 tablespoons fat-free sour cream; 2 tablespoons grated reduced-fat, natural Cheddar cheese or *2 tablespoons low-sodium, reduced-fat, natural Cheddar cheese*; and 1 tablespoon chopped scallions
1 cup green beans, cooked from frozen
1 small whole wheat roll with 1 teaspoon soft margarine or *1 teaspoon unsalted soft margarine*
1 small apple
1 cup fat-free milk

Snack
⅓ cup unsalted almonds
¼ cup raisins
1 cup orange juice

Nutritional Analysis
Total calories: 2,024; *1,998*
Total fat: 51 grams; *50 grams*
Sodium: 2,363 milligrams; *1,320 milligrams*

Day 2
Breakfast
½ cup instant flavored oatmeal or *½ cup regular oatmeal with 1 teaspoon cinnamon*
1 mini whole wheat bagel with 1 tablespoon fat-free cream cheese
1 medium banana
1 cup fat-free milk

Lunch
Chicken breast sandwich made with 2 slices (3 ounces) skinless chicken breast, 1 slice (¾ ounce) reduced-fat American cheese or *1 slice (¾ ounce) natural Swiss cheese*, 1 large leaf romaine lettuce, 2 slices tomato, 1 tablespoon low-fat mayonnaise, and 2 slices whole wheat bread
1 medium peach
1 cup apple juice

Dinner
1 cup spaghetti with ¾ cup Vegetarian Spaghetti Sauce (see page 131) or *6 ounces no-salt-added tomato paste and 3 tablespoons Parmesan cheese*
Spinach salad made with 1 cup fresh spinach leaves; ¼ cup grated fresh carrots; ¼ cup sliced fresh

mushrooms; ½ cup corn, cooked from frozen; ½ cup canned pears, juice pack; and 2 tablespoons Vinaigrette Salad Dressing (see page 130)

Snack
⅓ cup almonds
¼ cup dried apricots
1 cup no-sugar-added, fat-free fruit yogurt

Nutritional Analysis
Total calories: 1,977; *1,967*
Total fat: 60 grams; *59 grams*
Sodium: 2,152 milligrams; *1,577 milligrams*

Day 3
Breakfast
¾ cup wheat flakes cereal *or 2 cups puffed wheat cereal*
1 slice whole wheat bread with 1 teaspoon soft margarine *or 1 teaspoon unsalted soft margarine*
1 medium banana
1 cup fat-free milk
1 cup orange juice

Lunch
Beef barbecue sandwich made with 2 ounces eye of round beef, 1 tablespoon barbecue sauce, 2 slices (1 ½ ounces) reduced-fat Cheddar cheese *or 2 slices (1 ½ ounces) natural Swiss cheese*, 1 large leaf romaine lettuce, 2 slices tomato, and 1 sesame roll
1 cup New Potato Salad (see page 124)
1 medium orange

Dinner
3 ounces cod with 1 teaspoon lemon juice
½ cup long-grain brown rice

½ cup spinach, cooked from frozen
I small cornbread muffin *or I small white dinner roll*
with I teaspoon soft margarine *or I teaspoon unsalted
soft margarine*

Snack
I cup no-sugar-added, fat-free fruit yogurt
¼ cup dried fruit
2 large graham cracker rectangles with I tablespoon
reduced-fat peanut butter *or I tablespoon unsalted peanut butter*

Nutritional Analysis
Total calories: 1,984; *1,958*
Total fat: 44 grams; *46 grams*
Sodium: 2,303 milligrams; *1,519 milligrams*

Day 4
Breakfast
¾ cup cornflakes *or ½ cup corn grits with I teaspoon
unsalted, fat-free margarine*
½ cup no-sugar-added, fat-free fruit yogurt
I medium apple
I cup grape juice
I cup fat-free milk

Lunch
Sandwich made with 2 ounces low-sodium, low-fat
smoked ham *or 2 ounces low-fat roast beef;* I slice (¾
ounce) reduced-fat, natural Cheddar cheese; I large
leaf romaine lettuce; 2 slices tomato; I tablespoon
low-fat mayonnaise; and 2 slices whole wheat bread
I cup carrot sticks

Dinner

Chicken and Spanish Rice; *substitute 4 ounces no-salt-added tomato sauce in recipe* (see page 163)

½ cup green peas, cooked from frozen

1 small whole wheat roll with 1 teaspoon soft margarine *or 1 teaspoon unsalted soft margarine*

1 cup cantaloupe

1 cup fat-free milk

Snack

⅓ cup unsalted almonds

½ cup fruit cocktail

1 cup apple juice

Nutritional Analysis

Total calories: 2,011; *2,050*

Total fat: 51 grams; *52 grams*

Sodium: 2,259 milligrams; *1,441 milligrams*

Day 5

Breakfast

¾ cup frosted shredded wheat

2 slices whole wheat bread with 1 teaspoon soft margarine *or 1 teaspoon unsalted soft margarine* and 2 teaspoons no-sugar-added jelly

1 medium banana

1 cup orange juice

1 cup fat-free milk

Lunch

Salad plate with ½ cup Tuna Salad (see page 128); 1 large leaf romaine lettuce; 6 fat-free wheat crackers *or 2 unsalted, fat-free wheat crackers*; ½ cup 2% cottage

cheese or ½ cup unsalted 2% cottage cheese; and 1 cup canned pineapple, juice pack
4 small celery sticks
2 tablespoons fat-free ranch dressing or 2 tablespoons fat-free yogurt dressing

Dinner
3 ounces Turkey Meatloaf (see page 162) with 1 tablespoon ketchup or 2 teaspoons ketchup
1 small baked potato topped with 1 teaspoon soft margarine or 1 teaspoon unsalted soft margarine, 1 tablespoon low-fat sour cream, and 1 chopped scallion stalk
1 cup collard greens, cooked from frozen
1 medium peach
1 cup fat-free milk

Snack
½ medium bagel with 1 tablespoon reduced-fat peanut butter or 1 tablespoon unsalted, reduced-fat peanut butter
½ cup no-sugar-added, fat-free fruit yogurt

Nutritional Analysis
Total calories: 1,947; 1,941
Total fat: 38 grams; 40 grams
Sodium: 2,495 milligrams; 1,493 milligrams

Day 6
Breakfast
1 low-fat granola bar
1 medium banana
1 cup no-sugar-added, fat-free fruit yogurt

1 cup orange juice
1 cup fat-free milk

Lunch
Turkey breast sandwich made with 3 ounces turkey breast; 2 slices (1½ ounces) reduced-fat, natural Cheddar cheese *or 2 slices (1½ ounces) low-sodium, reduced-fat, natural Cheddar cheese*; 1 large leaf romaine lettuce; 2 slices tomato; 2 teaspoons low-fat mayonnaise; 1 tablespoon Dijon mustard *or 1 teaspoon regular mustard*; and 2 slices whole wheat bread
1 cup broccoli, steamed from frozen
1 medium orange

Dinner
3 ounces Spicy Baked Fish (see page 164)
1 cup Scallion Rice (see page 146)
½ cup spinach, cooked from frozen
1 cup carrots, cooked from frozen
1 small whole wheat roll with 1 teaspoon soft margarine *or 1 teaspoon unsalted soft margarine*
1 cup fat-free milk

Snack
2 large rectangle graham crackers *or 3 unsalted rice cakes*
¼ cup dried apricots
1 cup fat-free milk

Nutritional Analysis
Total calories: 1,944; *1,927*
Total fat: 31 grams; *28 grams*
Sodium: 2,331 milligrams; *1,568 milligrams*

Day 7
Breakfast
1 cup whole grain oat-rings cereal *or ½ cup regular oatmeal with 1 teaspoon cinnamon*
1 medium banana
1 cup no-sugar-added, fat-free fruit yogurt
1 cup fat-free milk

Lunch
Tuna salad sandwich made with ½ cup drained and rinsed tuna, 1 tablespoon low-fat mayonnaise, 1 large leaf romaine lettuce, 2 slices tomato, and 2 slices whole wheat bread
1 medium apple
1 cup fat-free milk

Dinner
⅙ recipe Zucchini Lasagna; *substitute unsalted cottage cheese in recipe* (see page 158)
Salad made with ½ cup fresh spinach leaves, ½ cup tomato wedges, 2 tablespoons seasoned croutons *or 2 tablespoons plain croutons*, and 2 tablespoons reduced-fat vinaigrette dressing *or 2 tablespoons Vinaigrette Salad Dressing (see page 130)*
1 small whole wheat roll with 1 teaspoon soft margarine *or 1 teaspoon unsalted soft margarine*
1 cup grape juice

Snack
⅓ cup unsalted almonds
2 slices (1½ ounces) reduced-fat, natural Cheddar cheese
6 whole wheat crackers

Nutritional Analysis
Total calories: 1,980; *1,966*
Total fat: 60 grams; *56 grams*
Sodium: 2,471 milligrams; *1,498 milligrams*

CHAPTER NINE

Recipes to Rein in Blood Pressure

If you think a diagnosis of high blood pressure means a life sentence to bland, boring—albeit healthy—foods, you're in for a delicious surprise. The collection of recipes in this chapter can shave points from your blood pressure reading without sacrificing taste or satisfaction. You'll reduce your risk of serious illness and maybe drop some extra pounds to boot!

We've chosen these particular recipes because they offer a smorgasbord of therapeutic nutrients, including potassium, which is linked to lower blood pressure and a reduced risk of stroke; calcium, another mineral shown to reduce blood pressure; and omega-3 fatty acids, "good" fats that improve blood pressure while decreasing the risk of heart disease. You'll also get plenty of fiber, which is good for your heart and your waistline.

What you won't be getting is a lot of sodium. These recipes supply no more than modest amounts. Instead, they get their palate-pleasing flavors from liberal amounts of herbs and spices.

You'll notice that a few of the recipes have an asterisk (*) beside their names. These correspond to specific menus in Chapter 8. Keep in mind that if you substitute any other recipe for one of the meal suggestions in the menu plan, your day's calorie, fat, and sodium intakes will change.

BREAKFASTS

Apple Skillet Cake

1 tablespoon butter
4 apples, peeled and sliced
2 tablespoons packed brown sugar
1/2 teaspoon ground cinnamon
1/2 cup raisins
3/4 cup whole grain pastry flour
1/3 cup sugar
1/8 teaspoon salt
1 1/2 cups 1% milk
2 eggs
1 egg white
2 teaspoons vanilla extract

Preheat the oven to 375°F.

In a medium ovenproof skillet, melt the butter over medium-high heat. Add the apples and cook for 2 minutes. Add the brown sugar, cinnamon, and raisins. Cook, stirring, for 5 minutes, or until the apples are tender. Remove from the heat and spread the apples evenly over the bottom of the skillet.

Meanwhile, in a large bowl, combine the flour, sugar, and salt.

In a medium bowl, combine the milk, eggs, egg white, and vanilla extract. Add to the flour mixture and stir just until blended. Pour over the apple mixture in the skillet.

Bake for 40 minutes, or until golden brown and puffed.

Remove to a rack to cool for 5 minutes. To serve, cut into wedges.

Makes 6 servings

Per serving: 279 calories, 5 g total fat, 2 g saturated fat, 79 mg cholesterol, 5 g dietary fiber, 147 mg sodium

Oat-Berry Pancakes with Vanilla-Ricotta Cream Sauce

Sauce

2 teaspoons cornstarch
1 cup orange juice
1 tablespoon lime juice
1 tablespoon honey

Ricotta Cream

⅔ cup fat-free ricotta cheese
2 tablespoons fat-free cream cheese
1 tablespoon honey
Grated peel of 1 lime
1 teaspoon vanilla extract

Pancakes

1 cup oat bran
1 cup whole grain pastry flour
1½ teaspoons baking powder
½ teaspoon baking soda
3 egg whites
2 cups buttermilk
2 cups mixed berries

To make the sauce: Place the cornstarch in a cup. Add 2 tablespoons of the orange juice and stir until smooth.

Place the remaining orange juice in a small saucepan. Add the lime juice and honey and cook, stirring constantly, over medium heat for 1 minute, or until the honey is dissolved.

Add the cornstarch mixture. Cook, stirring constantly, for 1 minute, or until thickened. Remove from the heat and set aside to cool. Cover and refrigerate for at least 3 hours before serving.

To make the ricotta cream: In a food processor or blender, process the ricotta until smooth. Add the cream cheese, honey, lime peel, and vanilla extract. Process until smooth. Refrigerate until ready to use.

To make the pancakes: Preheat the oven to 200°F. Coat a baking sheet with cooking spray.

In a large bowl, combine the oat bran, flour, baking powder, and baking soda.

In a medium bowl, combine the egg whites and buttermilk. Add to the flour mixture and stir just until blended.

Heat a large nonstick skillet coated with cooking spray over medium heat. For each pancake, spoon about 3 tablespoons batter into the skillet and spread to form a 3" pancake. Cook for 2 minutes, or until tiny bubbles appear on the surface and the edges begin to look dry. Flip and cook for 2 minutes, or until golden. Place the pancakes on the prepared baking sheet and place in the oven to keep warm. Repeat with the remaining batter to make a total of 8 pancakes.

For each serving, spread a pancake with the ricotta cream and top with a second pancake. Drizzle with the sauce and top with the berries.

Makes 4 servings

Per serving: 370 calories, 4 g total fat, 1 g saturated fat, 9 mg cholesterol, 10 g dietary fiber, 602 mg sodium

Sweet Potato Waffles

2¼ cups peeled and diced sweet potatoes
1½ cups light soy milk
3 egg whites
1 tablespoon canola oil

1 cup all-purpose flour
½ cup whole wheat flour
1 tablespoon baking powder
½ cup maple syrup
Raspberries and figs (optional)

Steam the sweet potatoes for 10 minutes, or until very soft. Transfer to a large bowl, and mash well. Beat in the milk, egg whites, and oil until smooth.

In a small bowl, whisk together the all-purpose flour, whole wheat flour, and baking powder. Pour over the liquid ingredients, and stir until smooth.

Heat a waffle iron, and lightly brush the grids with oil. For each waffle, pour in about ½ cup of batter, and spread it over the grids. Bake according to the manufacturer's directions.

Serve the waffles with the syrup, and top with raspberries and figs, if using.

Makes 8 servings
Per serving: 220 calories, 3 g total fat, 0 g saturated fat, 0 mg cholesterol, 3 g dietary fiber, 230 mg sodium

Florentine Omelette
2 eggs
2 egg whites
3 tablespoons water
1 teaspoon dried Italian seasoning, crushed
¼ teaspoon salt
8 ounces mushrooms, sliced
1 onion, chopped
1 red bell pepper, chopped
1 clove garlic, minced
4 ounces (2 packed cups) spinach leaves, chopped
¾ cup (3 ounces) shredded soy mozzarella cheese

Preheat the oven to 200°F. Coat a baking sheet with cooking spray.

In a medium bowl, whisk together the eggs, egg whites, water, Italian seasoning, and salt.

Coat a large nonstick skillet with cooking spray, and place over medium-high heat. Add the mushrooms, onion, pepper, and garlic. Cook, stirring often, for 4 minutes, or until the pepper starts to soften. Add the spinach, and cook for 1 minute, or until the spinach is wilted. Place in a small bowl, and cover.

Wipe the skillet with a paper towel. Coat with cooking spray, and place over medium heat. Pour in half of the egg mixture. Cook for 2 minutes, or until the bottom begins to set. Using a spatula, lift the edges to allow the uncooked mixture to flow to the bottom of the pan. Cook for 2 minutes longer, or until set. Sprinkle with half of the reserved vegetable mixture and half of the cheese. Cover, and cook for 2 minutes, or until the cheese melts. Using a spatula, fold the egg mixture in half. Place on the prepared baking sheet, and place in the oven to keep warm.

Coat the skillet with cooking spray. Repeat with the remaining egg mixture, vegetable mixture, and cheese to cook another omelette. To serve, cut each omelette in half.

Makes 4 servings

Per serving: 83 calories, 3 g total fat, 1 g saturated fat, 105 mg cholesterol, 3 g dietary fiber, 280 mg sodium

SOUPS

Cold Tomato and Cucumber Soup

2 pounds tomatoes, peeled and cut into chunks
1 large clove garlic
1 large cucumber, peeled, halved, seeded, and finely chopped
1 cup tomato juice

½ cup finely chopped fresh basil
1 tablespoon extra-virgin olive oil
1 tablespoon red wine vinegar
½ teaspoon salt
¼ teaspoon freshly ground black pepper

In 2 batches in a food processor, process the tomatoes and garlic until smooth. Place in a bowl.

Add the cucumber, tomato juice, basil, oil, vinegar, salt, and pepper to the bowl. Cover and chill for at least 3 hours, or until very cold and the flavors have blended.

Makes 4 servings
Per serving: 100 calories, 4 g total fat, 1 g saturated fat, 0 mg cholesterol, 3 g dietary fiber, 410 mg sodium

Cold Beet Borscht

1½ pounds beets, peeled and quartered
3½ cups vegetable broth
1 cup water
2 tablespoons lemon juice
1 tablespoon red wine vinegar
1 small cucumber, peeled and finely chopped
3 tablespoons reduced-fat sour cream
1 tablespoon snipped fresh dill

In a large saucepan or Dutch oven over high heat, combine the beets, broth, and water. Bring to a boil. Reduce the heat to low, cover, and simmer for 30 minutes, or until the beets are very tender.

With a slotted spoon, place the beets in a large bowl and allow them to cool to room temperature. Pour the cooking liquid into another large bowl and refrigerate.

Finely chop the cooled beets and add to the cooking liquid. Cover and refrigerate until cold.

Add the lemon juice and vinegar to the soup. Place half

of the soup in a blender or food processor and blend or process until smooth. Return the puree to the soup and add the cucumber.

Ladle the soup into bowls. In a cup, combine the sour cream and dill. Dollop onto each serving.

Makes 6 servings
Per serving: 67 calories, 1 g total fat, 1 g saturated fat, 3 mg cholesterol, 4 g dietary fiber, 484 mg sodium

Curried Sweet Potato and Apple Soup

1 tablespoon olive oil
1 large onion, sliced
2 cloves garlic, sliced
1 tablespoon finely chopped fresh ginger
1 teaspoon curry powder
3/4 teaspoon ground cumin
1/2 teaspoon salt
1/4 teaspoon ground cinnamon
4 cups water
1 1/4 pounds sweet potatoes, peeled and cut into chunks
3 large Granny Smith apples, peeled, cored, and cut into chunks
1/2 cup chopped fresh cilantro

In a large saucepan or Dutch oven, heat the oil over medium heat. Add the onion and garlic and cook, stirring occasionally, for 5 minutes, or until tender.

Add the ginger, curry powder, cumin, salt, and cinnamon. Cook, stirring constantly, for 1 minute. Add the water, sweet potatoes, and apples and bring to a boil over high heat. Reduce the heat to low, cover, and simmer, stirring often, for 20 minutes, or until the sweet potatoes are very tender.

In a food processor or blender, puree the soup in batches

until very smooth, pouring each batch into a bowl. Reheat if necessary. Stir in the cilantro.

Makes 8 servings

Per serving: 134 calories, 2 g total fat, 0 g saturated fat, 0 mg cholesterol, 4 g dietary fiber, 162 mg sodium

Turnip and Carrot Soup with Parmesan

1 pound white turnips, peeled and cut into chunks
4 large carrots, cut into chunks
2 large red or white new potatoes, peeled and cut into chunks
1 large onion, cut into chunks
5 cloves garlic, sliced
1 ½ cups chicken broth
1 ½ cups water
½ teaspoon dried thyme, crushed
½ teaspoon rubbed sage
¼ teaspoon salt
¼ teaspoon freshly ground black pepper
1 cup 1% milk
½ cup (2 ounces) freshly grated Parmesan cheese

In a large saucepan or Dutch oven, combine the turnips, carrots, potatoes, onion, garlic, broth, water, thyme, sage, salt, and pepper. Bring to a boil over high heat. Reduce the heat to medium, cover, and simmer for 20 minutes, or until the vegetables are very tender.

In a food processor or blender, puree the soup in batches until very smooth, pouring each batch into a bowl. When all the soup has been pureed, return it to the saucepan. Stir in the milk. Cook over low heat just until heated through (do not boil). Remove from the heat and stir in the cheese.

Makes 8 servings

Per serving: 108 calories, 2 g total fat, 1 g saturated fat, 6 mg cholesterol, 3 g dietary fiber, 364 mg sodium

Minestrone Verde

2 teaspoons extra-virgin olive oil
2 small leeks, white and green parts, halved lengthwise,
   rinsed, and thinly sliced
2 large ribs celery with leaves, thinly sliced
2 cloves garlic, minced + 1 whole clove garlic, peeled
1/4 teaspoon dried oregano, crushed
1/4 teaspoon freshly ground black pepper
1/8 teaspoon salt
2 cups water
1 cup chicken broth
4 cups chopped Swiss chard
2/3 cup frozen baby lima beans
1/4 cup ditalini or other small pasta
1/4 cup chopped Italian parsley
1/2 cup frozen green peas
4 teaspoons shredded Parmesan cheese

Heat the oil in a large saucepan over medium heat. Add the
leeks, celery, minced garlic, oregano, pepper, and salt. Cook,
stirring frequently, for 4 minutes, or until the vegetables begin to soften.

Add the water, broth, Swiss chard, lima beans, and pasta.
Bring to a boil over high heat. Reduce the heat to medium-
low, cover, and simmer for 8 minutes, or until the vegetables
are tender and the pasta is al dente.

Meanwhile, coarsely chop the remaining garlic clove, then
mince it together with the parsley. Stir the garlic-parsley
mixture and the peas into the soup. Cover and cook for 5
minutes, or until the peas are heated through.

Ladle the soup into 4 bowls and top each with 1 teaspoon
of the cheese.

Makes 4 servings
Per serving: 145 calories, 3 g total fat, 1 g saturated fat, 1 mg
cholesterol, 5 g dietary fiber, 413 mg sodium

Gingery Vegetable Broth with Tofu and Noodles

1 tablespoon canola oil

8 ounces cremini mushrooms, finely chopped

2 large carrots, finely chopped

2 ribs celery, finely chopped

1 medium onion, finely chopped

6 large cloves garlic, minced

2 tablespoons finely chopped fresh ginger

3 tablespoons dry sherry

4 cups low-sodium vegetable broth

1/4 teaspoon salt

1 cup snow peas, cut into julienne strips

4 ounces thin soba noodles, broken in half

8 ounces baked smoked tofu, cut into 1/4" cubes

4 scallions, thinly sliced on the diagonal

Heat the oil in a large saucepan or Dutch oven over medium-high heat. Add the mushrooms, carrots, celery, onion, garlic, and ginger. Cook, stirring often, for 10 minutes, or until the vegetables are lightly browned.

Add the sherry and cook for 1 minute, stirring to loosen browned bits from the pan. Add the broth and salt and bring to a boil over high heat. Reduce the heat to low, cover, and simmer for 45 minutes, adding the snow peas during the last 3 minutes.

Meanwhile, prepare the soba noodles according to package directions. Drain and set aside.

Stir the tofu, soba noodles, and scallions into the broth and simmer for 3 minutes, or until heated through.

Makes 4 servings

Per serving: 297 calories, 8 g total fat, 2 g saturated fat, 5 mg cholesterol, 6 g dietary fiber, 575 mg sodium

Black Bean Soup

2 cans (14–19 ounces each) black beans, rinsed and drained

1¾ cups low-sodium chicken broth

1 cup water

1 teaspoon ground cumin

¼ teaspoon dried oregano, crushed

¼ teaspoon freshly ground black pepper

Large pinch of ground red pepper

1 teaspoon olive oil

½ large red bell pepper, slivered

½ large green bell pepper, slivered

½ teaspoon grated lemon peel

In a large saucepan, combine the beans, broth, water, cumin, oregano, black pepper, and ground red pepper. Bring to a boil over high heat. Reduce the heat to low, cover, and simmer, stirring once or twice, for 15 minutes, or until the flavors are blended.

Meanwhile, heat the oil in a small nonstick skillet over medium heat. Add the bell peppers and cook, stirring frequently, for 4 minutes, or until tender.

Ladle half of the soup into a food processor or blender. Process or blend until pureed. Return the puree to the saucepan; add the lemon peel.

Ladle the soup into bowls and top each serving with the bell peppers.

Makes 4 servings

Per serving: 188 calories, 2 g total fat, 1 g saturated fat, 2 mg cholesterol, 14 g dietary fiber, 616 mg sodium

Cooking tip: To make this soup with dried beans, place 1 pound of beans in a large pot with cold water to cover and let sit overnight. Drain, cover with fresh water, and simmer for 1¼ hours, or until tender. You'll have enough for this recipe, plus leftovers for other dishes.

Tortilla Soup with Lime

4 corn tortillas (6" diameter), halved and cut into ¼"-wide strips

2¼ cups chicken broth

1¼ cups water

12 ounces thinly sliced turkey breast cutlets, cut into ½"-thick strips

2 large onions, halved and thinly sliced

2 large red bell peppers, cut into thin strips

1 large jalapeño chile pepper, seeded and minced (wear plastic gloves when handling)

2 teaspoons ground cumin

¼ teaspoon dried oregano, crushed

½ cup frozen corn kernels

½ cup quartered cherry tomatoes

¼ cup chopped fresh cilantro

2 tablespoons lime juice

½ ripe avocado, diced

Preheat the oven to 400°F. Coat 1 or 2 large baking sheets with cooking spray.

Arrange the tortilla strips on the prepared baking sheets and bake for 2 minutes, or until crisped and lightly browned on the edges.

In a large saucepan, combine the broth, water, turkey, onions, bell peppers, chile pepper, cumin, and oregano. Bring to a boil over high heat. Reduce the heat to medium-low, cover, and simmer for 10 minutes.

Add the corn and simmer for 5 minutes. Stir in the tomatoes, cilantro, and lime juice. Ladle the soup into bowls and top each portion with avocado and tortilla crisps.

Makes 4 servings

Per serving: 258 calories, 6 g total fat, 1 g saturated fat, 53 mg cholesterol, 6 g dietary fiber, 419 mg sodium

Split Pea Soup with Ham and Winter Squash

1 smoked ham hock (12 ounces)
11 cups water
4 cloves garlic, minced
1 teaspoon dried thyme, crushed
½ teaspoon dried sage, crushed
½ teaspoon freshly ground black pepper
1 pound green split peas, picked over and rinsed
1 medium butternut squash (2 pounds), peeled and cut into ½" chunks
1 pound white potatoes, scrubbed and cut into ½" chunks
3 large carrots, cut into ½" chunks
3 ribs celery, sliced
2 large onions, coarsely chopped
¾ teaspoon salt

In a large saucepan or Dutch oven, combine the ham hock, water, garlic, thyme, sage, and pepper. Bring to a boil over high heat. Reduce the heat to low, cover, and simmer for 1 hour, turning the ham hock once. Cool. Refrigerate for at least 4 hours or overnight.

After the broth has chilled, skim and discard the fat from the surface. Remove the ham hock. Cut the meat off the bone and set aside. Discard the bone and any fat.

Add the split peas to the broth and bring to a boil over high heat. Skim off any foam that rises to the surface. Reduce the heat to low, cover, and simmer, stirring occasionally, for 1 hour, or until the peas are soft and tender.

Add the squash, potatoes, carrots, celery, onions, salt, and ham. Return to a boil. Cover and simmer, stirring occasionally, for 20 to 25 minutes, or until the vegetables are tender.

Makes 8 servings

Per serving: 350 calories, 3 g total fat, 1 g saturated fat, 7 mg cholesterol, 19 g dietary fiber, 464 mg sodium

Root Vegetable Soup

1 tablespoon olive oil
6 cloves garlic, minced
2 large onions, chopped
½ teaspoon dried marjoram, crushed
½ teaspoon dried sage, crushed
¼ teaspoon salt
½ teaspoon freshly ground black pepper
1 pound lean, well-trimmed beef round, cut into 1" cubes
3 cups low-sodium beef broth
3 cups water
1 can (28 ounces) whole tomatoes, drained and broken up
4 small turnips, peeled and cut into ½" chunks
3 medium beets, peeled and cut into ½" chunks
3 large carrots, cut into ½" chunks
2 medium parsnips, peeled and cut into ½" chunks

In a large saucepan, heat the oil over medium heat. Add the garlic and onions and cook, stirring, for 5 minutes, or until soft. Add the marjoram, sage, salt, and pepper. Add the beef and cook, stirring, for 5 minutes, or until browned.

Add the broth, water, and tomatoes. Bring to a boil over high heat. Reduce the heat to low, cover, and simmer, stirring occasionally, for 45 minutes, or until the beef is very tender.

Add the turnips, beets, carrots, and parsnips. Return to a simmer. Cover and cook, stirring occasionally, for 25 minutes more, or until the vegetables are very tender.

Makes 6 servings

Per serving: 311 calories, 7 g total fat, 2 g saturated fat, 36 mg cholesterol, 9 g dietary fiber, 583 mg sodium

Creamy White Bean Soup with Cabbage and Salmon

1 cup navy beans, picked over, rinsed, and soaked overnight
2½ cups water
2 cups chicken broth
6 cloves garlic, minced
1 bay leaf
2 tablespoons extra-virgin olive oil
½ head cabbage, coarsely chopped
1 large onion, chopped
½ pound skinned salmon fillet, cut into 1" chunks
2 ounces (2 thick slices) Canadian bacon, coarsely chopped
1 tablespoon chopped fresh thyme

In a large saucepan or Dutch oven, combine the beans, water, broth, garlic, and bay leaf. Bring to a boil over high heat. Reduce the heat to low, cover, and simmer, stirring occasionally, for 50 minutes, or until the beans are very tender. Remove and discard the bay leaf.

In a food processor or blender, puree the soup in batches until smooth. Return the soup to the saucepan and bring to a boil over medium heat. Cover to keep warm.

Meanwhile, heat 1 tablespoon of the oil in a large nonstick skillet over high heat. Add the cabbage and onion. Cook, stirring frequently, for 6 minutes, or until lightly browned and tender. Add to the soup.

In the same skillet, heat the remaining 1 tablespoon oil over medium heat. Add the salmon and bacon. Sprinkle with the thyme. Cook, stirring gently, for 3 minutes, or until the salmon is lightly browned and just opaque.

Gently stir the salmon mixture into the soup.

Makes 4 servings
Per serving: 340 calories, 10 g total fat, 2 g saturated fat, 37 mg cholesterol, 14 g dietary fiber, 536 mg sodium

Manhattan Clam Chowder

2 teaspoons olive oil
2 ribs celery with leaves, chopped
2 carrots, chopped
1 onion, finely chopped
1 small clove garlic, minced
1 large potato, peeled and diced
1 green bell pepper, chopped
1 red bell pepper, chopped
¾ cup bottled clam juice
2 cans (6½ ounces each) chopped clams, drained with
    juice reserved
2½ cups reduced-sodium stewed tomatoes
1 teaspoon dried thyme, crushed
¼ teaspoon freshly ground black pepper
2–3 drops hot-pepper sauce

In a large saucepan or Dutch oven, heat the oil over medium heat. Add the celery, carrots, onion, and garlic. Cook, stirring, for 5 minutes, or until the onion is tender.

Add the potato, bell peppers, bottled clam juice, and the reserved clam juice. Bring to a boil. Reduce the heat to low, cover, and simmer, stirring, for 10 minutes, or until the potato is tender.

Add the tomatoes (with juice), thyme, black pepper, hot-pepper sauce, and the reserved clams. Bring to a simmer. Cover and simmer for 8 minutes, or until the flavors are blended.

Makes 4 servings
Per serving: 138 calories, 3 g total fat, 1 g saturated fat, 17 mg cholesterol, 4 g dietary fiber, 754 mg sodium

Chunky Chicken Chili

2 tablespoons olive oil

4 cloves garlic, minced

2 jalapeño or serrano chile peppers, partially seeded, and minced (wear plastic gloves when handling)

1 large onion, chopped

1 pound fresh tomatillos, husked, rinsed, and coarsely chopped (see cooking tip)

2 teaspoons ground cumin

1/2 teaspoon salt

1/4 teaspoon freshly ground black pepper

1 1/2 cups chicken broth

1 pound boneless, skinless chicken breasts, cut into 3/4" cubes

2 cups frozen cut leaf spinach (from a bag)

1 can (15 1/2 ounces) whole hominy, drained and rinsed

1/2 cup chopped fresh cilantro

Heat the oil in a large saucepot or Dutch oven over medium heat. Add the garlic, chile peppers, and onion. Cook, stirring frequently, for 8 minutes, or until soft.

Stir in the tomatillos, cumin, salt, and pepper. Reduce the heat to low, cover, and cook, stirring frequently, for 5 minutes, or until the tomatillos are softened.

Stir in the broth, chicken, spinach, and hominy. Bring to a boil over high heat. Reduce the heat to low and cook, stirring occasionally, for 5 minutes, or until the chicken is no longer pink.

Stir in the cilantro.

Makes 6 servings

Per serving: 237 calories, 7 g total fat, 1 g saturated fat, 44 mg cholesterol, 6 g dietary fiber, 662 mg sodium

Cooking tip: Tomatillos are Mexican green tomatoes. Smaller than their red tomato cousins, they are often sold with a papery husk. Remove and discard the husk before using.

Fish Stew with Couscous

2 cloves garlic, minced
1 onion, halved and thinly sliced
1 teaspoon ground cumin
1/4 teaspoon ground cinnamon
1 can (15 ounces) chopped tomatoes
1 can (14–19 ounces) chickpeas, rinsed and drained
1 cup chicken broth
1/3 cup pitted prunes, chopped
1/4 cup halved pitted kalamata olives
4 orange roughy or halibut fillets (4 ounces each)
1 box (10 ounces) couscous

Coat a large nonstick skillet with cooking spray. Add the garlic, onion, cumin, and cinnamon. Coat lightly with cooking spray and place over medium heat. Cook, stirring, for 8 minutes, or until the onion is soft.

Add the tomatoes, chickpeas, broth, prunes, and olives. Cook, stirring occasionally, for 5 minutes. Push the mixture to the edges of the skillet. Add the fish. Spoon the chickpea mixture over the fish. Cover, reduce the heat to low, and cook for 10 minutes, or until the fish flakes easily.

Meanwhile, cook the couscous according to package directions. Fluff with a fork. Evenly divide among 4 plates and top with the fish and chickpea mixture.

Makes 4 servings

Per serving: 576 calories, 5 g total fat, 0 g saturated fat, 23 mg cholesterol, 12 g dietary fiber, 680 mg sodium

Pasta e Fagiole

2 teaspoons olive oil
2 onions, chopped
2 cloves garlic, chopped
4 cups low-sodium chicken broth
1 can (15 ounces) diced tomatoes

2 cans (14–19 ounces each) cannellini or white beans,
    rinsed and drained
1/2 cup ditalini or other small pasta
4 cups chopped Swiss chard or spinach

In a large saucepan, heat the oil over medium heat. Add the
onions and garlic and cook, stirring occasionally, for 5
minutes, or until the onions are soft.

Add the broth, tomatoes (with juice), beans, and pasta
and cook, stirring occasionally, for 15 minutes, or until the
pasta is al dente. Add the Swiss chard or spinach and cook,
stirring occasionally, for 3 minutes, or until the chard or
spinach is wilted.

Makes 6 servings
Per serving: 186 calories, 3 g total fat, 1 g saturated fat, 3 mg
cholesterol, 5 g dietary fiber, 584 mg sodium

SALADS

Southwestern Quinoa and Chickpea Salad
1 cup quinoa (see cooking tip)
1 3/4 cups water
1/8 teaspoon salt
1 cup rinsed and drained canned chickpeas
1 medium tomato, seeded and chopped
1 clove garlic, minced
3 tablespoons lime juice
2 tablespoons finely chopped fresh cilantro
4 teaspoons olive oil
1/2 teaspoon ground cumin

Place the quinoa in a fine-mesh strainer and rinse under cold
running water until the water runs clear.

In a medium saucepan, bring the water to a boil over high
heat. Add the quinoa and salt and return to a boil. Reduce

the heat to low, cover, and simmer for 20 minutes, or until tender and the liquid is absorbed.

Meanwhile, in a large bowl, combine the chickpeas, tomato, garlic, lime juice, cilantro, oil, and cumin. Add the quinoa and toss to coat well.

Makes 4 servings

Per serving: 283 calories, 8 g total fat, 1 g saturated fat, 0 mg cholesterol, 6 g dietary fiber, 200 mg sodium

Cooking tip: You must thoroughly rinse quinoa to remove the saponin, a naturally occurring coating on the grain that has a bitter flavor.

Kamut, Orange, and Fennel Salad

1 cup whole grain kamut, spelt, or wheat berries
2½ cups water
1 cup chicken or vegetable broth
3 medium navel oranges
2 tablespoons extra-virgin olive oil
1 tablespoon balsamic vinegar
½ teaspoon salt
¼ teaspoon freshly ground black pepper
1 medium bulb fennel, chopped
1 large red bell pepper, chopped
1 small red onion, chopped
¼ cup sliced pitted kalamata olives

Place the kamut, spelt, or wheat berries in a sieve and rinse until the water runs clear. Place in a bowl with 2 cups of the water. Let stand for 8 hours or overnight. Drain.

Place the kamut, spelt, or wheat berries, the remaining ½ cup water, and the broth in a medium saucepan and bring to a boil over high heat. Reduce the heat to low, cover, and simmer for 45 minutes, or until tender and some of the grains have burst.

Drain in a colander and place in a medium bowl. Let stand for 30 minutes, or until cooled.

Cut off the peel and most of the white membrane from two of the oranges. Cut each orange in half through the top end and place the half flat on a cutting board. Cut the half lengthwise into ½" slices. Juice the remaining orange. In a small bowl, whisk together the orange juice, oil, vinegar, salt, and black pepper.

Add the fennel, bell pepper, onion, and olives to the ka-mut, spelt, or wheat berries. Add the orange juice mixture and toss to coat well. Add the oranges and toss gently.

Serve immediately or cover and chill to serve later.

Makes 8 servings
Per serving: 149 calories, 5 g total fat, 1 g saturated fat, 0 mg cholesterol, 5 g dietary fiber, 272 mg sodium

Mediterranean Chickpea Salad

1 can (15 ounces) chickpeas, rinsed and drained
3 plum tomatoes, chopped
2 roasted red peppers, chopped
½ small red onion, quartered and thinly sliced
½ cucumber, peeled, halved, seeded, and chopped
2 tablespoons chopped parsley
2 cloves garlic, chopped
3 tablespoons lemon juice
1½ teaspoons extra-virgin olive oil
1½ teaspoons flaxseed oil
¼ teaspoon salt

In a large bowl, combine the chickpeas, tomatoes, peppers, onion, cucumber, parsley, garlic, lemon juice, olive oil, flaxseed oil, and salt. Toss to coat well. Let stand for at least 15 minutes to allow the flavors to blend.

Makes 8 servings

Per serving: 104 calories, 3 g total fat, 0 g saturated fat, 0 mg cholesterol, 4 g dietary fiber, 158 mg sodium

Wheat Berry Salad

1 cup wheat berries or whole grain spelt
3½ cups water
2 cups chicken or vegetable broth
3 cups small broccoli florets
2 tablespoons extra-virgin olive oil
2 cloves garlic, minced
1 tablespoon fresh herb, such as basil, rosemary, or marjoram, or 1 teaspoon dried, crushed
2 cups halved mixed red and yellow cherry tomatoes
1 cup fresh, drained canned, or frozen corn kernels
¼ teaspoon salt
¼ teaspoon freshly ground black pepper

Place the wheat berries or spelt in a sieve and rinse until the water runs clear. Place in a bowl with 2 cups of the water. Let stand for 8 hours or overnight. Drain.

Place the remaining 1½ cups water and broth in a medium saucepan and bring to a boil over high heat. Add the wheat berries or spelt and return to a boil. Reduce the heat to low, cover, and simmer for 45 minutes, adding the broccoli during the last 5 minutes. Drain and place in a large bowl.

Meanwhile, heat the oil in a skillet over medium-high heat. Add the garlic and herb and cook, stirring, for 1 minute. Add the tomatoes, corn, salt, and pepper and cook, stirring frequently, for 3 minutes, or until the tomatoes begin to collapse. Serve over the wheat berries or spelt.

Makes 6 servings
Per serving: 256 calories, 9 g total fat, 1 g saturated fat, 0 mg cholesterol, 12 g dietary fiber, 460 mg sodium

Asian Slaw

1/4 cup rice wine vinegar or white wine vinegar
2 tablespoons soy sauce
1 tablespoon grated fresh ginger
2 teaspoons toasted sesame oil
1/2 head napa or savoy cabbage, shredded
3 scallions, sliced
2 carrots, shredded
1/2 red bell pepper, cut into thin strips
2 tablespoons chopped fresh cilantro
2 teaspoons sesame seeds, toasted (optional)

In a large bowl, combine the vinegar, soy sauce, ginger, and oil. Add the cabbage, scallions, carrots, pepper, and cilantro. Toss to coat well. Sprinkle with the sesame seeds, if using. Let stand for at least 15 minutes to allow the flavors to blend.

Makes 4 servings

Per serving: 106 calories, 3 g total fat, 0 g saturated fat, 0 mg cholesterol, 5 g dietary fiber, 561 mg sodium

Roasted Beet Salad

4 medium beets (about 1 pound), stems trimmed to 1"
2 tablespoons apricot all-fruit spread
1 tablespoon white balsamic vinegar
1 1/2 teaspoons olive oil
1 1/2 teaspoons flaxseed oil
2 tablespoons snipped fresh chives or thinly sliced scallion
    greens
1/2 teaspoon salt
1/4 teaspoon freshly ground black pepper
2 medium navel oranges
4 cups mixed bitter salad greens, such as arugula, water-
    cress, endive, and escarole

Preheat the oven to 400°F. Coat a 9" baking pan with cooking spray.

Place the beets in the prepared baking pan and cover tightly with foil. Roast for 1 hour, or until very tender. Uncover and let the beets stand until cool enough to handle.

Meanwhile, in a large bowl, whisk the all-fruit spread, vinegar, olive oil, flaxseed oil, chives or scallions, salt, and pepper.

Slip the skins off the beets and discard the skins. Chop the beets. Cut off the peel and white pith from the oranges. Section the oranges into the bowl with the dressing. Add the beets and toss to coat well. Let stand for at least 15 minutes to allow the flavors to blend.

Just before serving, arrange the greens on a serving plate. Top with the beet mixture.

Makes 4 servings

Per serving: 144 calories, 4 g total fat, 0 g saturated fat, 0 mg cholesterol, 5 g dietary fiber, 390 mg sodium

Potato Salad with Warm Onion Dressing

2 pounds red potatoes, cut into large chunks
1 tablespoon canola oil
1 large red onion, chopped
1 clove garlic, chopped
3 tablespoons cider vinegar
3 tablespoons apple juice
1 tablespoon stone-ground mustard
¼ cup chopped parsley
⅛ teaspoon salt

Place a steamer basket in a saucepan with ½" of water. Place the potatoes in the steamer. Bring to a boil over high heat. Reduce the heat to medium, cover, and cook for 20 minutes, or until tender. Rinse briefly under cold running water and drain. Place in a large serving bowl.

Meanwhile, heat the oil in a medium nonstick skillet over medium heat. Add the onion and garlic and cook, stirring, for 8 minutes, or until the onion is very soft.

Add the vinegar, apple juice, mustard, parsley, and salt. Cook for 2 minutes, or until heated through. Pour over the potatoes. Toss to coat well. Let stand for at least 15 minutes to allow the flavors to blend.

Makes 6 servings

Per serving: 145 calories, 3 g total fat, 0 g saturated fat, 0 mg cholesterol, 3 g dietary fiber, 103 mg sodium

New Potato Salad*

16 small new potatoes, scrubbed
2 tablespoons olive oil
¼ cup green onions, chopped
¼ teaspoons freshly ground black pepper
1 teaspoon dried dillweed

Place the potatoes in a large saucepan and add just enough water to cover the potatoes. Bring to a boil over high heat. Reduce the heat, cover, and cook for 20 minutes, or until tender. Drain and cool the potatoes for 20 minutes.

Cut the potatoes into fourths and transfer to a large bowl. Add the olive oil, onions, pepper, and dillweed and toss to coat well. Refrigerate before serving.

Makes 5 servings

Per serving: 187 calories, 6 g total fat, 1 g saturated fat, 0 mg cholesterol, 3 g dietary fiber, 12 mg sodium

Roasted Sweet-Potato Salad

2 tablespoons olive oil
¼ teaspoon salt
¼ teaspoon freshly ground black pepper
2 pounds sweet potatoes, scrubbed and cut into 1" chunks
2 large red bell peppers, cut into 1" pieces

  2 tablespoons white balsamic or white wine vinegar
  1 pound spinach or arugula, torn into bite-size pieces

Preheat the oven to 425°F.

In a large roasting pan, combine the oil, salt, and black pepper. Add the sweet potatoes and bell peppers and toss to coat well. Roast, stirring occasionally, for 40 minutes, or until the potatoes are tender. Remove from the oven and stir in the vinegar.

Place the spinach or arugula in a large serving bowl. Add the potato mixture and toss to coat well. Serve immediately.

Makes 4 servings

Per serving: 336 calories, 8 g total fat, 1 g saturated fat, 0 mg cholesterol, 18 g dietary fiber, 312 mg sodium

Grilled Steak and Potato Salad
Steak and Vegetables
  1 pound well-trimmed boneless beef top sirloin or top round steak, about 1" thick
  4 cloves garlic, minced
  ½ teaspoon coarsely ground black pepper
  ¼ teaspoon salt
  1 large red onion, cut into ½"-thick slices, rings separated
  1 teaspoon extra-virgin olive oil
  1 teaspoon red wine vinegar
  8 small red or white new potatoes, scrubbed and halved

Salad
  2½ teaspoons red wine vinegar
  2 teaspoons extra-virgin olive oil
  2 teaspoons flaxseed oil
  1½ teaspoons coarse Dijon mustard
  1 teaspoon water
  1 small clove garlic, minced
  ¼ teaspoon freshly ground black pepper

⅛ teaspoon salt
1 package (5 ounces) mesclun leaves or baby greens

To make the steak and vegetables: Coat a grill rack or broiler-pan rack with cooking spray. Preheat the grill or broiler.

Rub the steak on both sides with the garlic, pepper, and salt, pressing them into the surface. Place on one side of the prepared rack. On a plate, toss the onion with the oil and vinegar and place the onion on the other side of the rack. Let stand for 5 minutes.

Meanwhile, place a steamer basket in a saucepan with ½" of water. Place the potatoes in the steamer. Bring to a boil over high heat. Reduce the heat to medium, cover, and cook for 7 minutes, or until fork-tender.

Grill or broil the steak and onion for 6 minutes, turning once, or until a thermometer inserted in the center of the steak registers 145°F for medium-rare. Remove the steak to a plate. Let stand for 10 minutes, then slice. Continue grilling or broiling the onion rings, turning frequently, for 4 minutes longer, or until tender and lightly charred.

To make the salad: In a large bowl, whisk together the vinegar, olive oil, flaxseed oil, mustard, water, garlic, pepper, and salt until well-blended. Add the greens, potatoes, onion, steak, and any accumulated meat juices. Toss to coat well.

Makes 4 servings

Per serving: 273 calories, 9 g total fat, 2 g saturated fat, 49 mg cholesterol, 3 g dietary fiber, 326 mg sodium

Thai Rice and Turkey Salad

1 cup brown basmati rice
½ cup water
½ cup chicken broth
1 tablespoon grated fresh ginger
2 cloves garlic, minced

12 ounces boneless, skinless turkey breast, cut crosswise
    into strips
3 tablespoons smooth natural peanut butter
3 tablespoons lime juice
1 teaspoon honey
1/4 teaspoon salt
2 cups shredded napa cabbage
1 large red bell pepper, finely chopped
1 small red onion, finely chopped
3 tablespoons coarsely chopped fresh mint
3 cups small tender spinach or kale leaves
2 tablespoons coarsely chopped roasted, unsalted peanuts

Prepare the rice according to package directions. Spread the rice in a shallow baking pan and place it in the freezer for 10 minutes to chill slightly.

Meanwhile, place the water, broth, ginger, and garlic in a medium skillet. Bring to a boil over high heat. Reduce the heat to low, cover, and simmer for 5 minutes. Add the turkey, cover, and cook, stirring frequently, for 4 minutes, or until the turkey is no longer pink. Using a slotted spoon, remove the turkey to a plate. Cover loosely with waxed paper to keep it moist.

Increase the heat to high and return the broth to a boil. Boil for 6 minutes, or until the broth is thickened and reduced to about 1/4 cup.

In a large bowl, whisk together the peanut butter, lime juice, honey, and salt. Whisk in the reduced broth and continue whisking until smooth (add a few drops of hot water if the mixture becomes too thick). Add the rice, turkey and any accumulated juices, cabbage, pepper, onion, and mint. Toss to coat well.

Arrange the spinach or kale on a platter. Mound the salad in the center and sprinkle with the peanuts.
Makes 4 servings

Per serving: 408 calories, 9 g total fat, 2 g saturated fat, 53 mg cholesterol, 7 g dietary fiber, 295 mg sodium

Chicken Salad*
3¼ cups cooked, diced skinless chicken
¼ cup chopped celery
1 tablespoon lemon juice
½ teaspoon onion powder
⅛ teaspoon salt (see note)
3 tablespoons low-fat mayonnaise

Refrigerate the cooked chicken.

In a large bowl, combine the celery, lemon juice, onion powder, salt, and mayonnaise. Add the chilled chicken and toss to coat well.

Makes 5 servings
Per serving: 183 calories, 7 g total fat, 2 g saturated fat, 78 mg cholesterol, 0 g dietary fiber, 201 mg sodium
Health note: To reduce the sodium content of this recipe, you can leave out the salt.

Tuna Salad*
2 cans (6 ounces each) water-packed tuna
½ cup chopped celery
⅓ cup chopped scallions
6½ tablespoons reduced-fat mayonnaise

Rinse and drain the tuna for 5 minutes. In a medium bowl, break apart tuna with a fork. Add the celery, scallions, and mayonnaise, and mix well.

Makes 5 servings
Per serving: 146 calories, 7 g total fat, 0 g saturated fat, 25 mg cholesterol, 1 g dietary fiber, 158 mg sodium

Pasta Salad with Shrimp and Broccoli

8 ounces small pasta shells
1½ cups broccoli florets
1 medium carrot, sliced
1 red bell pepper, sliced
1 tablespoon olive oil
2 cloves garlic, minced
1 scallion, minced
12 ounces shrimp, peeled, deveined, and sliced lengthwise
in half
1 large tomato, chopped
½ cup buttermilk
2 tablespoons red wine vinegar
1 tablespoon flaxseed oil
1 tablespoon Dijon mustard
1 teaspoon freshly ground black pepper
½ teaspoon salt

Prepare the pasta according to package directions, adding the broccoli, carrot, and bell pepper during the last 5 minutes of cooking.

Meanwhile, heat the olive oil in a large skillet over medium heat. Add the garlic and scallion and cook for 1 minute. Add the shrimp and cook, stirring frequently, for 3 minutes, or until the shrimp are opaque. Add the tomato and cook for 1 minute. Remove from the heat.

Meanwhile, in a large bowl, combine the buttermilk, vinegar, flaxseed oil, mustard, black pepper, and salt. Add the shrimp mixture and pasta mixture and toss to coat well.

Makes 8 servings
Per serving: 205 calories, 5 g total fat, 1 g saturated fat, 65 mg cholesterol, 2 g dietary fiber, 244 mg sodium

DRESSINGS AND SAUCES

Yogurt Salad Dressing*
8 ounces fat-free plain yogurt
1/4 cup fat-free mayonnaise
2 tablespoons dried chives
2 tablespoons dried dillweed
2 tablespoons lemon juice

In a small bowl, combine the yogurt, mayonnaise, chives, dillweed, and lemon juice. Refrigerate.
Makes 8 servings
Per serving: 23 calories, 0 g total fat, 0 g saturated fat, 1 mg cholesterol, 0 g dietary fiber, 84 mg sodium

Vinaigrette Salad Dressing*
1 bulb garlic, separated and peeled
1/2 cup water
1 tablespoon red wine vinegar
1 tablespoon virgin olive oil
1/4 teaspoon honey
1/4 teaspoon freshly ground black pepper

Place the garlic cloves in a small saucepan and pour in enough water (about 1/2 cup) to cover them. Bring the water to a boil, then reduce the heat and simmer for about 15 minutes, or until the garlic is tender.

Reduce the liquid to 2 tablespoons and increase the heat for 3 minutes. Pour the contents into a small sieve over a bowl and, with a wooden spoon, mash the garlic through the sieve. Whisk the vinegar into the garlic mixture; mix in the oil, honey, and pepper.
Makes 4 servings

Per serving: 33 calories, 3 g total fat, 1 g saturated fat, 0 mg cholesterol, 0 g dietary fiber, 0 mg sodium

Vegetarian Spaghetti Sauce*

2 tablespoons olive oil
2 small onions, chopped
3 cloves garlic, chopped
1 ¼ cups sliced zucchini
1 tablespoon dried oregano
1 tablespoon dried basil
1 can (8 ounces) tomato sauce
1 can (6 ounces) tomato paste (see note)
2 medium tomatoes, chopped
1 cup water

Heat the oil in a medium skillet over medium heat. Add the onions, garlic, and zucchini and cook, stirring frequently, for 5 minutes, or until tender.

Add the oregano, basil, tomato sauce, tomato paste, tomatoes, and water. Simmer covered for 45 minutes. Serve over spaghetti.

Makes 6 servings

Per serving: 102 calories, 5 g total fat, 1 g saturated fat, 0 mg cholesterol, 5 g dietary fiber, 459 mg sodium

Health note: To reduce the sodium content of this recipe, use a 6-ounce can of no-salt-added tomato paste.

VEGETABLE SIDE DISHES

Stuffed Acorn Squash

3 acorn squash, halved lengthwise and seeded
⅔ cup quick-cooking barley
2 teaspoons vegetable oil
1 small onion, chopped

   1 rib celery, chopped
   1 clove garlic, chopped
   3 ounces mushrooms, sliced
   1/4 cup chopped fresh parsley and/or thyme or sage or 2
        teaspoons dried, crushed
   1 cup coarse fresh bread crumbs
   2/3 cup dried cranberries
   1 teaspoon grated lemon peel
   1/4 teaspoon salt
   1/4–1/2 cup vegetable broth or apple juice

Preheat the oven to 400°F.

Place the squash, cut side up, on a baking sheet. Coat the cut sides lightly with cooking spray. Bake for 30 minutes, or until fork-tender.

Meanwhile, prepare the barley according to package directions.

Heat the oil in a medium nonstick skillet over medium heat. Add the onion, celery, and garlic and cook for 2 minutes. Add the mushrooms and parsley and/or thyme or sage and cook for 4 minutes, or until the mushrooms are soft. Remove from the heat. Stir in the bread crumbs, cranberries, lemon peel, salt, and barley. Add up to 1/2 cup broth or apple juice to moisten and bind the stuffing.

Reduce the oven temperature to 350°F. Spoon the stuffing into the squash halves. Bake for 10 minutes, or until heated through.

Makes 6 servings

Per serving: 198 calories, 3 g total fat, 0 g saturated fat, 0 mg cholesterol, 6 g dietary fiber, 190 mg sodium

Cooking tip: Ingredients for savory recipes should be considered options, not dictates. If you don't care for an ingredient in the list, feel free to make substitutions. Any number of grains can take the place of barley in Stuffed Acorn Squash, for example. Try quinoa, millet, cracked wheat berries, or even chunks of whole grain bread. Instead of cranberries, use dried cherries, dried apricots, diced apples, diced pears, or another fresh or dried fruit of your choice. By tailoring recipes to suit your tastes, a healthy eating plan is sure to succeed.

Sweet-and-Sour Red Cabbage and Apples

1 tablespoon butter
1 tablespoon canola oil
1 large onion, chopped
½ medium head red cabbage, cored and shredded
½ teaspoon salt
¼ teaspoon freshly ground black pepper
¼ teaspoon ground allspice
3 medium sweet-tart apples (such as Golden Delicious),
    peeled, cored, and cut into thin wedges
¼ cup frozen apple juice concentrate
2 tablespoons red wine vinegar

In a large saucepot or Dutch oven, heat the butter and oil over medium heat until the butter melts. Add the onion and cook, stirring frequently, for 6 minutes, or until soft.

Add the cabbage, salt, pepper, and allspice. Cook, stirring frequently, for 4 minutes, or until the cabbage begins to wilt and the color starts to change.

Add the apples, apple juice concentrate, and vinegar. Bring to a boil. Reduce the heat to low, cover, and simmer, stirring frequently, for 15 minutes, or until the cabbage is very tender.

Makes 6 servings
Per serving: 124 calories, 5 g total fat, 1 g saturated fat, 5 mg cholesterol, 4 g dietary fiber, 235 mg sodium

Roasted Beets with Herbs and Garlic

2 pounds small beets, scrubbed
2 tablespoons chicken or vegetable broth
1 tablespoon extra-virgin olive oil
2 cloves garlic, minced
1 large shallot, finely chopped
½ teaspoon dried sage, crushed
Pinch of ground allspice
⅛ teaspoon salt
⅛ teaspoon freshly ground black pepper

Preheat the oven to 400°F.

Cut each beet into 8 wedges. Place the beets, broth, oil, garlic, shallot, sage, allspice, salt, and pepper in an 11" × 7" baking dish. Toss to coat well.

Cover tightly with foil and bake, stirring occasionally, for 1 hour, or until the beets are very tender.

Makes 4 servings
Per serving: 132 calories, 4 g total fat, 1 g saturated fat, 0 mg cholesterol, 5 g dietary fiber, 288 mg sodium

Roasted Garlic

1 large bulb garlic
Pinch of salt

Preheat the oven to 400°F.

Cut a thin slice from the top of the garlic to expose the cloves. Place the head, cut side up, on a large piece of foil. Seal the top and sides of the foil tightly. Place in the oven and roast for 35 minutes, or until the cloves are very soft and lightly browned. Remove and set aside until cool enough to handle.

Squeeze the garlic cloves into a small bowl. With the back of a spoon, mash the garlic with the salt to make a smooth paste. Use in place of butter on potatoes, rice, or bread.

Makes 4 tablespoons

Per 2 tablespoons: 22 calories, 0 g total fat, 0 g saturated fat, 0 mg cholesterol, 0 g dietary fiber, 94 mg sodium

Health note: Although garlic isn't loaded with vitamins and minerals, it is brimming with phytochemicals. You'll get the most by eating your garlic raw, but only one phytochemical is lost in cooking, so eat as much garlic as possible, both raw and cooked.

Stuffed Vidalia Onions

4 Vidalia or sweet onions
½ teaspoon olive oil
2 medium zucchini, shredded
3 cloves garlic, minced
1 teaspoon dried thyme, crushed
1 teaspoon dried basil, crushed
3 tablespoons plain dry bread crumbs
1½ tablespoons chopped toasted pine nuts
3 tablespoons freshly grated Parmesan cheese
¼ teaspoon salt
¼ teaspoon freshly ground black pepper

Preheat the oven to 400°F. Line a small baking pan with foil.

Cut ½" off the top of each onion. Slightly trim the bottoms so that the onions stand upright. Place the onions, cut side up, in the prepared baking pan and coat with cooking spray. Bake for 1 hour, or until soft. Set aside for 15 minutes, or until cool enough to handle.

Reduce the oven temperature to 350°F.

Remove and discard the onion peels. Using a spoon, scoop out the onion centers, leaving a ½" shell. Chop the centers and reserve 1 cup for the stuffing. Save the remainder for another use.

Heat the oil in a large nonstick skillet over medium heat.

Add the zucchini, garlic, thyme, basil, and the 1 cup chopped onion. Cook for 6 minutes, or until the zucchini is softened and most of the liquid has evaporated. Remove from the heat and stir in the bread crumbs, pine nuts, 2½ tablespoons of the cheese, salt, and pepper.

Divide the filling among the onion shells. Place the onion shells in the same baking pan and top with the remaining ½ tablespoon cheese.

Bake for 20 minutes, or until golden.

Makes 4 servings

Per serving: 122 calories, 4 g total fat, 1 g saturated fat, 3 mg cholesterol, 4 g dietary fiber, 262 mg sodium

Roasted Carrots and Parsnips

1 pound carrots, cut into 1" chunks
1 pound parsnips, cut into 1" chunks
4 small red onions, cut into wedges
6 cloves garlic
½ tablespoon olive oil
½ teaspoon salt
½ teaspoon grated lemon peel

Preheat the oven to 375°F. Coat a medium baking pan with cooking spray. Add the carrots, parsnips, onions, garlic, oil, salt, and lemon peel. Toss to coat well.

Bake, stirring occasionally, for 40 minutes, or until golden and tender.

Makes 6 servings

Per serving: 113 calories, 2 g total fat, 0 g saturated fat, 0 mg cholesterol, 7 g dietary fiber, 229 mg sodium

Grilled Portobellos, Peppers, and Onions

¼ cup chopped flat-leaf parsley
3 tablespoons lemon juice
2 tablespoons extra-virgin olive oil

3 cloves garlic, minced

1 teaspoon dried Italian herb seasoning, crushed

1/2 teaspoon freshly ground black pepper

1/4 teaspoon salt

2 large red bell peppers, cut into strips

6 ounces portobello mushrooms, sliced

1 large sweet white onion, halved and cut into 1"-thick slices

Coat a grill rack with cooking spray. Preheat the grill to medium-hot.

In a large bowl, combine the parsley, lemon juice, oil, garlic, Italian seasoning, black pepper, and salt. Add the bell peppers, mushrooms, and onion and toss to coat well. (The mixture can be prepared ahead to this point and refrigerated up to 2 days.)

Place a vegetable basket or grill screen on the grill rack and place the vegetables on the basket or screen. Grill, turning often, for 15 minutes, or until very tender and lightly charred.

Makes 4 servings

Per serving: 110 calories, 7 g total fat, 1 g saturated fat, 0 mg cholesterol, 3 g dietary fiber, 155 mg sodium

Cooking tip: To cook this dish indoors, coat a broiler-pan rack with cooking spray and preheat the broiler. Place the vegetables on the rack and broil, turning often, for 10 minutes, or until browned.

Stewed Vegetables

2 teaspoons extra-virgin olive oil

1 large onion, halved and thinly sliced

3 cloves garlic, thinly sliced

1 can (16 ounces) whole tomatoes

1/2 teaspoon dried thyme, crushed

1/4 teaspoon salt

1 pound green beans, halved
1 medium zucchini, halved lengthwise and thinly sliced
1/2 cup fresh basil leaves, cut into thin strips

Heat the oil in a large nonstick skillet over medium heat. Add the onion and garlic and cook, stirring occasionally, for 4 minutes, or until tender.

Add the tomatoes (with juice), thyme, and salt, stirring to break up the tomatoes. Bring to a boil over high heat. Add the green beans. Reduce the heat to low, cover, and simmer, stirring occasionally, for 10 minutes, or until the beans are tender.

Add the zucchini and cook, stirring occasionally, for 5 minutes, or until tender. Remove from the heat and stir in the basil.

Makes 4 servings
Per serving: 95 calories, 3 g total fat, 0 g saturated fat, 0 mg cholesterol, 6 g dietary fiber, 465 mg sodium

Artichoke Gratin

2 packages (9 ounces each) frozen artichoke hearts
1 tablespoon lemon juice
3 tablespoons plain dry bread crumbs
1 tablespoon freshly grated Parmesan cheese
1 teaspoon dried Italian herb seasoning, crushed
1 clove garlic, minced
1 teaspoon olive oil

Preheat the oven to 375°F. Coat a 9" glass pie plate with cooking spray.

Place the artichokes in a colander and rinse well with cold water to separate. Drain well, then pat dry with paper towels. Place in the prepared pie plate and sprinkle with the lemon juice.

In a small bowl, combine the bread crumbs, cheese, Italian seasoning, garlic, and oil. Sprinkle the mixture evenly over the artichokes.

Bake for 15 minutes, or until the topping is golden.

Makes 4 servings

Per serving: 102 calories, 2 g total fat, 0 g saturated fat, 1 mg cholesterol, 7 g dietary fiber, 184 mg sodium

Stir-Fried Asparagus with Ginger, Sesame, and Soy

1½ pounds thin asparagus, cut diagonally into 2" pieces
2 teaspoons canola oil
½ large red bell pepper, cut into thin strips
1 tablespoon chopped fresh ginger
1 tablespoon reduced-sodium soy sauce
⅛ teaspoon crushed red-pepper flakes
1 teaspoon toasted sesame oil
1 teaspoon sesame seeds, toasted

Bring ¼" water to a boil in a large nonstick skillet over high heat. Add the asparagus and return to a boil. Reduce the heat to low, cover, and simmer for 5 minutes, or until crisp-tender. Drain in a colander and cool briefly under cold running water. Wipe the skillet dry with a paper towel.

Heat the canola oil in the same skillet over high heat. Add the bell pepper and cook, stirring constantly, for 3 minutes, or until crisp-tender. Add the asparagus, ginger, soy sauce, and red-pepper flakes and cook for 2 minutes, or until heated through. Remove from the heat and stir in the sesame oil and sesame seeds.

Makes 4 servings

Per serving: 79 calories, 5 g total fat, 0 g saturated fat, 0 mg cholesterol, 4 g dietary fiber, 157 mg sodium

Braised Italian Peppers with Onions and Thyme

1 tablespoon extra-virgin olive oil

6–8 Italian frying peppers, cut into 2" chunks

1 large red onion, cut into wedges

1 tablespoon balsamic vinegar

2 teaspoons coarsely chopped fresh thyme or ¼ teaspoon dried, crushed

⅛ teaspoon salt

⅛ teaspoon freshly ground black pepper

2 plum tomatoes, cut into ½" chunks

3 tablespoons chicken or vegetable broth or water

Heat the oil in a large skillet over medium heat. Add the frying peppers and onion and cook, stirring occasionally, for 5 minutes, or until the onion starts to soften.

Add the vinegar, thyme, salt, and black pepper and cook for 1 minute. Add the tomatoes and broth or water. Reduce the heat to low, cover, and simmer, stirring occasionally, for 8 minutes, or until the vegetables are very tender.

Makes 4 servings

Per serving: 90 calories, 4 g total fat, 1 g saturated fat, 0 mg cholesterol, 3 g dietary fiber, 134 mg sodium

Cauliflower with Red Pepper and Garlic

1 large head cauliflower, cut into small florets

1 large red bell pepper, cut into 1" squares

2 tablespoons extra-virgin olive oil

4 cloves garlic, minced

1 tablespoon red wine vinegar

2 teaspoons chopped fresh thyme or ¼ teaspoon dried, crushed

¾ teaspoon paprika

½ teaspoon salt

Place a steamer basket in a large saucepan with ½" of water. Place the cauliflower and pepper in the steamer. Bring to a boil over high heat. Reduce the heat to medium, cover, and cook for 4 minutes, or until crisp-tender. Place in a serving bowl.

Heat the oil in a small skillet over medium heat. Remove from the heat and stir in the garlic. When the sizzling stops, stir in the vinegar, thyme, paprika, and salt. Add to the vegetables and toss to coat well.

Makes 4 servings

Per serving: 122 calories, 7 g total fat, 1 g saturated fat, 0 mg cholesterol, 5 g dietary fiber, 345 mg sodium

Curried Cauliflower and Carrots with Beans

1 large head cauliflower, cut into small florets
2 large carrots, cut into ½"-thick diagonal slices
2 tablespoons olive oil
1 medium onion, chopped
1 tablespoon finely chopped fresh ginger
2 cloves garlic, minced
1 tablespoon unbleached all-purpose flour
1½–2 teaspoons curry powder
1 cup chicken or vegetable broth
2 tablespoons dry white wine
1 can (14–19 ounces) black beans or chickpeas, rinsed and drained
½ cup chopped fresh cilantro or flat-leaf parsley

Place a steamer basket in a large saucepan with ½" of water. Place the cauliflower and carrots in the steamer. Bring to a boil over high heat. Reduce the heat to medium, cover, and cook for 10 minutes, or until tender. Place in a bowl and keep warm. Rinse and dry the saucepan.

Heat the oil in the same saucepan over medium heat. Add

the onion, ginger, and garlic and cook, stirring frequently, for 3 minutes, or until soft.

In a cup, combine the flour and curry powder. Add to the saucepan and cook, stirring, for 1 minute.

Gradually stir in the broth and wine and bring to a boil. Reduce the heat to low and simmer, stirring frequently, for 5 minutes, or until the sauce is lightly thickened.

Add the beans or chickpeas and cook, stirring, for 3 minutes, or until heated through. Add to the vegetables in the bowl and toss gently just until combined. Sprinkle with the cilantro or parsley.

Makes 6 servings
Per serving: 140 calories, 5 g total fat, 1 g saturated fat, 0 mg cholesterol, 8 g dietary fiber, 281 mg sodium

Stir-Fried Broccoli and Mushrooms with Tofu

1/3 cup chicken or vegetable broth
1 tablespoon apricot all-fruit spread
1 tablespoon reduced-sodium soy sauce
1 tablespoon dry sherry
2 teaspoons cornstarch
1 tablespoon canola oil
1 large bunch broccoli, cut into small florets
4 cloves garlic, minced
1 tablespoon finely chopped fresh ginger
4 ounces mushrooms, sliced
1 cup halved cherry and/or yellow pear tomatoes
8 ounces firm tofu, drained and cut into 1/4" cubes

In a cup, whisk together the broth, all-fruit spread, soy sauce, sherry, and cornstarch. Set aside.

Heat the oil in a large nonstick skillet over medium-high heat. Add the broccoli, garlic, and ginger and cook, stirring constantly, for 1 minute. Add the mushrooms and cook, stirring frequently, for 3 minutes, or until crisp-tender and lightly browned.

Add the tomatoes and tofu and cook, stirring frequently, for 2 minutes, or until the tomatoes begin to collapse.

Stir the cornstarch mixture and add to the skillet. Cook, stirring, for 2 minutes, or until the mixture boils and thickens.

Makes 4 servings

Per serving: 147 calories, 7 g total fat, 1 g saturated fat, 0 mg cholesterol, 4 g dietary fiber, 230 mg sodium

Indian-Spiced Potatoes and Spinach

2 medium russet potatoes, scrubbed and cut into ½" chunks

2 tablespoons canola oil

3 large cloves garlic, minced

1 medium onion, chopped

1¾ teaspoons ground cumin

¾ teaspoon ground coriander

½ teaspoon ground turmeric

¼ teaspoon ground ginger

¼ teaspoon salt

¼ teaspoon freshly ground black pepper

⅛ teaspoon ground cinnamon

2 cups frozen cut leaf spinach (from a bag)

2–4 tablespoons water

½ cup (4 ounces) fat-free plain yogurt

Place a steamer basket in a large saucepan with ½" of water. Place the potatoes in the steamer. Bring to a boil over high heat. Reduce the heat to medium, cover, and cook for 20 minutes, or until the potatoes are very tender.

Place the potatoes in a bowl and keep warm. Drain and dry the saucepan.

Heat the oil in the same saucepan over medium heat. Add

the garlic and onion and cook, stirring frequently, for 5 minutes, or until soft. Add the cumin, coriander, turmeric, ginger, salt, pepper, and cinnamon and cook, stirring, for 30 seconds to cook the spices.

Add the potatoes and cook, stirring frequently, for 5 minutes, or until crisp and golden.

Add the spinach and 2 tablespoons water. Cover and cook, tossing gently, adding additional water 1 tablespoon at a time, if needed, for 5 minutes, or until heated through.

Place in a serving bowl. Spoon the yogurt on top, but don't stir it in, and serve hot.

Makes 4 servings

Per serving: 195 calories, 7 g total fat, 1 g saturated fat, 1 mg cholesterol, 6 g dietary fiber, 350 mg sodium

Fluffy Garlic Mashed Potatoes

4 medium russet or Yukon gold potatoes, cut into 1" chunks

8 cloves garlic

½ cup buttermilk

1 tablespoon butter

½ teaspoon salt

¼ teaspoon freshly ground black pepper

1 tablespoon snipped fresh chives, dill, or scallion greens   ·

Place a steamer basket in a large saucepan with ½" of water. Place the potatoes and garlic in the steamer. Bring to a boil over high heat. Reduce the heat to medium, cover, and cook for 20 minutes, or until the potatoes are very tender.

Place the potatoes and garlic in a bowl and mash with a potato masher. Add the buttermilk, butter, salt, pepper, and chives, dill, or scallion greens. Mash until well-blended.

Makes 4 servings

Per serving: 172 calories, 4 g total fat, 2 g saturated fat, 9 mg cholesterol, 3 g dietary fiber, 360 mg sodium

Spicy Oven Fries

2 medium russet potatoes, scrubbed and cut into long 1/4"-
   thick strips
1 tablespoon canola oil
1 tablespoon roasted garlic and red-pepper spice blend
1/4 teaspoon salt
1/4 teaspoon freshly ground black pepper

Preheat the oven to 425°F. Coat a 13" × 9" baking pan with
cooking spray.

Place the potatoes in a mound in the prepared baking pan
and sprinkle with the oil, spice blend, salt, and pepper. Toss
to coat well. Spread the potatoes in a single layer.

Bake, turning the potatoes several times, for 40 minutes,
or until crisp and lightly browned.

Makes 4 servings

Per serving: 115 calories, 4 g total fat, 0 g saturated fat, 0 mg
cholesterol, 2 g dietary fiber, 144 mg sodium

GRAIN SIDE DISHES

Cilantro and Tomato Rice

1 cup short-grain brown rice
2 cups water
1/2 teaspoon salt
1 pound tomatoes, coarsely chopped
1/3 cup chopped fresh cilantro
1 tablespoon extra-virgin olive oil
1 tablespoon lime juice or lemon juice
1 clove garlic, minced
1 teaspoon ground cumin
1/4 teaspoon freshly ground black pepper
1 can (14–19 ounces) chickpeas, rinsed and drained
1/4 cup slivered almonds, toasted

In a medium saucepan, place the rice, water, and ¼ teaspoon of the salt. Bring to a boil over high heat. Reduce the heat to low, cover, and simmer for 50 minutes, or until the rice is tender and the liquid is absorbed.

Meanwhile, in a medium bowl, combine the tomatoes, cilantro, oil, lime juice or lemon juice, garlic, cumin, pepper, and the remaining ¼ teaspoon salt. Cover and let stand at room temperature. Stir in the rice and chickpeas and top with the almonds.

Makes 4 servings
Per serving: 405 calories, 11 g total fat, 1 g saturated fat, 0 mg cholesterol, 10 g dietary fiber, 472 mg sodium

Scallion Rice*
4½ cups cooked rice
1½ teaspoons bouillon granules, unsalted
¼ cup scallions, chopped

Cook the rice in unsalted water according to directions on the package. Combine the cooked rice, bouillon granules, and scallions, and mix well. Measure 1-cup portions and serve.

Makes 5 servings
Per serving: 185 calories, 1 g total fat, 0 g saturated fat, 0 mg cholesterol, 1 g dietary fiber, 3 mg sodium

Millet Pilaf
1 cup millet
1½ cups water
1 cup chicken broth
¼ teaspoon salt
½ cup golden raisins
2 tablespoons dry sherry
1 tablespoon extra-virgin olive oil
⅓ cup natural almonds, coarsely chopped

1 ½ teaspoons chopped fresh rosemary
2 tablespoons chopped flat-leaf parsley

In a medium saucepan over medium-high heat, cook the millet, stirring frequently, for 4 minutes, or until the grains are fragrant, browned in spots, and just beginning to crackle.

Add the water, broth, and salt. Bring to a boil over high heat. Reduce the heat to low, cover, and simmer for 25 minutes, or until the millet is tender, some grains have burst, and the water has evaporated. Remove from the heat and let stand, covered, for 10 minutes.

Meanwhile, in a small bowl, soak the raisins in the sherry.

Heat the oil in a small skillet over medium heat. Add the almonds and cook, stirring frequently, for 4 minutes, or until lightly toasted. Stir in the rosemary and raisins and cook, stirring, for 30 seconds. Remove from the heat.

Fluff the millet with a fork. Stir in the almond mixture and sprinkle with the parsley.

Makes 4 servings

Per serving: 359 calories, 11 g total fat, 1 g saturated fat, 0 mg cholesterol, 7 g dietary fiber, 299 mg sodium

Polenta with Fresh Tomato Sauce
6 cups water
¾ teaspoon salt
2 cups coarse yellow cornmeal
½ cup (2 ounces) freshly grated Parmesan cheese
1 tablespoon extra-virgin olive oil
1 large clove garlic, minced
¼ teaspoon dried oregano, crushed
¼ teaspoon fennel seeds, crushed
8 plum tomatoes, coarsely chopped
⅛ teaspoon freshly ground black pepper
2 tablespoons tomato paste

Preheat the oven to 400°F. Coat a 9" × 9" baking dish with cooking spray.

Bring the water to a boil in a large saucepan over high heat. Stir in ½ teaspoon of the salt. Add the cornmeal in a slow, steady stream, whisking constantly. Bring to a boil. Stir in the cheese.

Remove from the heat and pour into the prepared baking dish. Bake for 35 minutes, or until firm.

Meanwhile, heat the oil in a large nonstick skillet over medium heat. Add the garlic, oregano, and fennel seeds and cook, stirring, for 3 minutes, or until fragrant.

Stir in the tomatoes, pepper, and the remaining ¼ teaspoon salt. Increase the heat to high and bring to a boil. Reduce the heat to medium-low and simmer, stirring frequently, for 8 minutes, or until the tomatoes are cooked down and juicy. Add the tomato paste and cook, stirring, for 2 minutes, or until the sauce is slightly thickened. Cover and keep warm.

Serve the polenta with the sauce.

Makes 6 servings

Per serving: 246 calories, 7 g total fat, 2 g saturated fat, 7 mg cholesterol, 5 g dietary fiber, 497 mg sodium

Garlic and Red Pepper Grits

3¾ cups water
½ teaspoon salt
¾ cup quick-cooking grits
1 tablespoon canola oil
3 cloves garlic, minced
2 large red bell peppers, chopped
½ teaspoon paprika
½ teaspoon dried thyme, crushed
¼ teaspoon freshly ground black pepper
⅓ cup (1½ ounces) shredded Monterey Jack cheese

In a medium saucepan, bring the water to a boil over high heat. Add the salt and slowly stir in the grits. Reduce the heat to medium-low and cook, stirring occasionally, for 20 minutes, or until the grits are creamy and thickened. Remove from the heat.

Meanwhile, in a medium nonstick skillet, heat the oil over medium-low heat. Add the garlic and cook, stirring, for 2 minutes, or until fragrant. Add the bell peppers, paprika, thyme, and black pepper and cook, stirring frequently, for 8 minutes, or until very tender. (Add a tablespoon of water to the pan if it gets dry.)

Stir the bell pepper mixture and the cheese into the grits, stirring until the cheese melts.

Makes 4 servings

Per serving: 185 calories, 7 g total fat, 2 g saturated fat, 10 mg cholesterol, 3 g dietary fiber, 358 mg sodium

Barley with Spring Greens

1 1/2 cups chicken or vegetable broth
1/2 cup pearl barley
1 tablespoon extra-virgin olive oil
1 bunch scallions, thinly sliced
3 cloves garlic, slivered
10 cups loosely packed torn mixed greens, such as escarole, Swiss chard, watercress, and arugula
1/4 teaspoon salt
1/8 teaspoon freshly ground black pepper

In a medium saucepan, bring the broth to a boil over high heat. Add the barley and return to a boil. Reduce the heat to low, cover, and simmer for 45 minutes, or until tender.

Meanwhile, in a large saucepot or Dutch oven, heat the oil over medium-high heat. Add the scallions and garlic and cook, stirring frequently, for 3 minutes, or until the scallions are wilted.

Add the greens, salt, and pepper. Cook, stirring, for 3 minutes, or until just wilted.

Fluff the barley with a fork and stir into the greens.

Makes 4 servings

Per serving: 143 calories, 4 g total fat, 1 g saturated fat, 0 mg cholesterol, 7 g dietary fiber, 391 mg sodium

Baked Barley with Mushrooms and Carrots

1 tablespoon butter
3 large carrots, halved lengthwise and thinly sliced
1 large onion, halved and thinly sliced
1 1/4 cups vegetable or chicken broth
10–12 ounces cremini, baby portobello, or white button
     mushrooms, sliced
2 cups water
1 cup pearl barley
1 teaspoon dried thyme, crushed
1/2 teaspoon salt
1/4 teaspoon freshly ground black pepper

Preheat the oven to 350°F.

Melt the butter in an ovenproof Dutch oven over medium-high heat. Add the carrots, onion, and 1 tablespoon of the broth. Cook, stirring frequently, for 8 minutes, or until tender, adding another 1 tablespoon broth halfway through cooking.

Add the mushrooms and 2 tablespoons of the remaining broth and cook, stirring frequently, for 4 minutes, or until tender.

Stir in the remaining 1 cup broth, the water, barley, thyme, salt, and pepper. Bring to a boil over high heat. Cover the pot and place in the oven. Bake for 45 minutes, or until the barley is tender and the liquid is absorbed.

Makes 6 servings

Per serving: 176 calories, 3 g total fat, 1 g saturated fat, 5 mg cholesterol, 8 g dietary fiber, 392 mg sodium

Quinoa with Peperonata

1 cup quinoa (see cooking tip)
2 cups water
½ teaspoon salt
2 tablespoons extra-virgin olive oil
3 large red bell peppers, cut into ½" squares
3 cloves garlic, minced
2 inner stalks celery with leaves, thinly sliced
1 medium red onion, chopped
¼ teaspoon freshly ground black pepper
1 can (14½ ounces) diced tomatoes, drained, with 2 tablespoons of the liquid reserved
2 strips orange peel (each 2" long), removed with a vegetable peeler
1 tablespoon drained capers, chopped

Place the quinoa in a fine-mesh strainer and rinse under cold running water until the water runs clear.

Place the water in a medium saucepan and bring to a boil over high heat. Add the quinoa and ¼ teaspoon of the salt and return to a boil. Reduce the heat to low, cover, and simmer for 20 minutes, or until the quinoa is tender and the water is absorbed.

Meanwhile, in a large skillet, heat the oil over medium heat. Add the bell peppers, garlic, celery, onion, black pepper, and the remaining ¼ teaspoon salt. Cook, stirring frequently, for 8 minutes, or until crisp-tender.

Stir in the tomatoes and the reserved 2 tablespoons tomato liquid, the orange peel, and capers. Bring to a boil over high heat. Reduce the heat to low, cover, and simmer, stirring occasionally, for 12 minutes, or until the vegetables are very tender. Remove and discard the orange peel.

Fluff the quinoa with a fork and spoon into a shallow serving dish. Top with the pepper mixture.

Makes 4 servings

Per serving: 262 calories, 10 g total fat, 1 g saturated fat, 0 mg cholesterol, 5 g dietary fiber, 605 mg sodium

Cooking tip: You must thoroughly rinse the quinoa to remove the saponin, a naturally occurring coating on the grain that has a bitter flavor.

Quinoa with Peppers and Beans

1 cup quinoa (see cooking tip)
2½ cups vegetable broth
2 tablespoons extra-virgin olive oil
3 cloves garlic, minced
1 tablespoon finely chopped peeled fresh ginger
¾ teaspoon whole cumin seeds
2 medium red bell peppers, cut into thin strips
1 large onion, cut into thin wedges
1 can (14–19 ounces) black beans, rinsed and drained
¼ cup chopped fresh cilantro

Place the quinoa in a fine-mesh strainer and rinse under cold running water until the water runs clear.

In a medium saucepan, bring 2 cups of the broth to a boil over high heat. Add the quinoa and return to a boil. Reduce the heat to low, cover, and simmer for 20 minutes, or until tender.

Meanwhile, in a large nonstick skillet, heat the oil over medium heat. Add the garlic, ginger, and cumin seeds and cook, stirring, for 2 minutes, or until fragrant. Add the peppers and onion and cook, stirring, for 8 minutes, or until tender. Stir in the beans and the remaining ½ cup broth and cook for 2 minutes.

Fluff the quinoa with a fork and stir in the cilantro. Place in a serving bowl and top with the pepper mixture.

Makes 4 servings
Per serving: 307 calories, 10 g total fat, 1 g saturated fat, 0
mg cholesterol, 9 g dietary fiber, 637 mg sodium
Cooking tip: You must thoroughly rinse the quinoa to remove
the saponin, a naturally occurring coating on the grain that
has a bitter flavor.

LEGUME SIDE DISHES

Soybeans with Sesame and Scallions

1 bag (12 ounces) frozen shelled green soybeans (eda-
   mame)
1 tablespoon soy sauce
½ cup water
1½ teaspoons sesame oil
Dash of hot-pepper sauce (optional)
2 tablespoons minced scallions
⅛ teaspoon freshly ground black pepper

In a medium saucepan over high heat, bring the soybeans,
soy sauce, and water to a boil, stirring occasionally. Reduce
the heat to low and simmer for 12 minutes, or until tender.
If any liquid remains, cook, stirring occasionally, over
medium-high heat until the liquid has evaporated.

Remove from the heat. Stir in the oil, hot-pepper sauce
(if using), scallions, and black pepper.

Makes 4 servings
Per serving: 132 calories, 5 g total fat, 0 g saturated fat, 0 mg
cholesterol, 5 g dietary fiber, 280 mg sodium

Adzuki Beans with Miso Dressing

1¼ cups dried adzuki beans, small red beans, or black
   beans, picked over and rinsed
¼ teaspoon freshly ground black pepper
2 tablespoons mellow white miso

   3 tablespoons orange juice
   2 tablespoons lemon juice
   2 tablespoons olive oil
   1/2 teaspoon grated fresh ginger
   3 scallions, diagonally sliced
   2 medium cucumbers, peeled, halved, seeded, and cut into
       thin diagonal slices
   1 small carrot, shredded
   1/4 cup coarsely chopped walnuts

Place the beans in a bowl. Add water to cover by 2". Cover
and let stand overnight.

Drain the beans and place in a medium saucepan. Add
water to cover by 2" and bring to a boil over high heat. Stir
in the pepper. Reduce the heat to low, cover, and simmer,
stirring, for 30 minutes, or until very tender.

Drain the beans and place in a serving bowl for 20
minutes.

Meanwhile, in a large bowl, whisk together the miso, orange juice, lemon juice, oil, and ginger. Stir in the scallions,
cucumbers, carrot, walnuts, and beans.

Let stand for 15 minutes to blend the flavors.

Makes 4 servings

Per serving: 351 calories, 12 g total fat, 2 g saturated fat, 0
mg cholesterol, 10 g dietary fiber, 327 mg sodium

Cooking tip: Though perfect as a main course, these hearty
beans are also well-suited as a side dish. Just halve the portions to get 8 tasty side-dish servings.

Lentils with Tomatoes

   1 1/2 cups brown lentils, picked over and rinsed
   3 1/2 cups water
   1/4 teaspoon ground allspice
   1/2 teaspoon freshly ground black pepper
   3/4 teaspoon salt

  2 tablespoons extra-virgin olive oil
  2 cloves garlic, minced
  3 medium tomatoes, cut into 1 1/2" chunks
  1/2 cup (4 ounces) fat-free plain yogurt
  2 tablespoons snipped fresh chives or scallion greens

In a large saucepan, combine the lentils, water, allspice, and 1/4 teaspoon of the pepper. Bring to a boil over high heat. Reduce the heat to low, cover, and simmer for 25 minutes, or until the lentils are tender but still hold their shape. Remove from the heat and stir in 1/2 teaspoon of the salt.

Meanwhile, in a large nonstick skillet, heat the oil over medium-high heat. Add the garlic and cook, stirring, for 30 seconds, or until fragrant. Add the tomatoes, the remaining 1/4 teaspoon salt, and the remaining 1/4 teaspoon pepper. Cook, stirring occasionally, for 2 minutes, or until the tomatoes just start to release their juices. Remove from the heat.

Drain the lentils and place in a shallow serving dish. Spoon the tomato mixture over the lentils, top with the yogurt, and sprinkle with the chives or scallion greens.

Makes 4 servings

Per serving: 344 calories, 8 g total fat, 1 g saturated fat, 1 mg cholesterol, 23 g dietary fiber, 482 mg sodium

Botana

  1 tablespoon olive oil
  5 cloves garlic, minced
  3/4 teaspoon ground cumin
  3/4 teaspoon dried oregano, crushed
  2 cans (14–19 ounces each) black beans, rinse and drain
      1 can, use both beans and liquid from other can
  1 can (15 ounces) diced tomatoes with green chiles
  1/4–1/2 cup water

½ cup (2 ounces) shredded reduced-fat sharp Cheddar
  cheese
Baked tortilla chips or warmed corn tortillas
Red bell pepper wedges, cucumber spears, and celery
  sticks for dipping

In a large nonstick skillet, heat the oil over medium heat.
Add the garlic, cumin, and oregano and cook, stirring frequently, for 2 minutes, or until fragrant.

Stir in the drained beans and the beans with their liquid
and bring to a boil. Remove from the heat. Mash the beans
with a potato masher to a coarse-textured puree.

Return to medium heat and stir in the tomatoes and ¼
cup of the water. Bring to a boil, stirring. Reduce the heat
to medium-low and cook, stirring frequently, for 5 minutes,
or until the beans are heated through and the flavors are
blended. Stir in up to ¼ cup additional water if the mixture
is too thick.

Place in a serving bowl and sprinkle with the cheese.
Serve with the chips or tortillas and vegetables.

Makes 8 servings
Per serving: 103 calories, 3 g total fat, 1 g saturated fat, 5 mg
cholesterol, 5 g dietary fiber, 494 mg sodium

SANDWICHES

Herbed Chicken Sandwiches
Lemon-Dill Mayonnaise
½ cup low-fat mayonnaise
1 teaspoon lemon juice
2 teaspoons chopped fresh basil or ½ teaspoon dried,
  crushed
2 teaspoons chopped fresh dill or ½ teaspoon dried,
  crushed

Sandwiches

12 thin slices multigrain bread, toasted
½ pound cooked skinless chicken breast, sliced
⅓ English cucumber, thinly sliced
1 large tomato, cut into 8 slices
1 cup mesclun or spring mix salad greens

To make the lemon-dill mayonnaise: In a small bowl, combine the mayonnaise, lemon juice, basil, and dill.

To make the sandwiches: Place 4 of the bread slices on a work surface. Spread 2 teaspoons of the lemon-dill mayonnaise on each slice. Top with layers of chicken and cucumber.

Spread 4 of the remaining bread slices each with 2 teaspoons of the lemon-dill mayonnaise. Place the bread, mayonnaise side up, on the 4 sandwiches. Top with layers of tomato and greens.

Spread the remaining 4 bread slices with the remaining lemon-dill mayonnaise. Place, mayonnaise side down, on top of the sandwiches. Cut in half diagonally and secure with wooden picks.

Makes 4 servings
Per serving: 375 calories, 11 g total fat, 2 g saturated fat, 56 mg cholesterol, 5 g dietary fiber, 587 mg sodium

Niçoise Salad Pockets
Dressing
½ cup balsamic or cider vinegar
1 tablespoon extra-virgin olive oil
1 tablespoon flaxseed oil
1 teaspoon Dijon mustard
1 teaspoon dried Italian seasoning, crushed
1 clove garlic, minced

Sandwiches

¾ pound red potatoes, cut into ¼"-thick slices

¼ pound small green beans

1 can (6 ounces) water-packed white tuna, drained and flaked

¼ red onion, thinly sliced

2 hard-cooked egg whites, coarsely chopped

¼ cup coarsely chopped niçoise olives

2 cups baby spinach leaves

4 whole wheat pitas, halved crosswise

To make the dressing: In a large bowl, combine the vinegar, olive oil, flaxseed oil, mustard, Italian seasoning, and garlic.

To make the sandwiches: Place a steamer basket in a saucepan with ½" of water. Place the potatoes and beans in the steamer. Bring to a boil over high heat. Reduce the heat to medium, cover, and cook for 7 minutes, or until crisptender. Rinse briefly under cold running water and drain.

To the bowl with the dressing, add the potatoes, beans, tuna, onion, egg whites, olives, and spinach. Toss to coat well.

Spoon the tuna mixture into each pita pocket. Drizzle lightly with any dressing left in the bowl.

Makes 4 servings

Per serving: 406 calories, 12 g total fat, 1 g saturated fat, 18 mg cholesterol, 9 g dietary fiber, 633 mg sodium

ENTRÉES

Zucchini Lasagna*

8 ounces lasagna noodles

¾ cup shredded reduced-fat mozzarella cheese

¼ cup freshly grated Parmesan cheese

1½ cups fat-free cottage cheese (see note)

1½ cups sliced zucchini

2½ cups no-salt-added tomato sauce
2 teaspoons dried basil
2 teaspoons dried oregano
¼ cup chopped onion
1 clove garlic, minced
⅛ teaspoon freshly ground black pepper

Preheat the oven to 350°F. Lightly coat a 13" × 9" baking dish with cooking spray and set aside.

Prepare the lasagna noodles according to package directions, using unsalted water.

Meanwhile, in a small bowl, combine ⅛ cup of the mozzarella and 1 tablespoon of the Parmesan. Set aside.

In a medium bowl, combine the cottage cheese with the remaining mozzarella and Parmesan. Mix well and set aside.

Combine the tomato sauce with the basil, oregano, onion, garlic, and pepper. Spread a thin layer of the tomato mixture in the bottom of the baking dish. Add one-third of the noodles in a single layer. Spread half of the cottage cheese mixture on top. Add a layer of zucchini. Repeat layering. Add a thin coating of sauce. Top with noodles, sauce, and reserved cheese mixture. Cover with aluminum foil.

Bake for 30 to 40 minutes. Cool for 10 to 15 minutes then cut into 6 portions.

Makes 6 servings
Per serving: 276 calories, 5 g total fat, 2 g saturated fat, 11 mg cholesterol, 5 g dietary fiber, 380 mg sodium
Health note: To reduce the sodium content of this recipe, use unsalted cottage cheese.

Penne with Salmon and Roasted Vegetables
12 ounces penne
2 pounds leeks
1 red bell pepper, cut into strips
¼ cup chicken broth

  2 tablespoons lemon juice
  1 tablespoon olive oil
  2 teaspoons dried thyme, crushed
  1/4 teaspoon freshly ground black pepper
  1 yellow summer squash, halved and cut into 1/4" slices
  1/4 cup pitted kalamata olives
  1 salmon fillet (1/2 pound), skinned

Preheat the oven to 400°F. Prepare the pasta according to package directions.

Meanwhile, cut the leeks into 2" lengths and quarter them lengthwise. Rinse the leeks completely. Place the leeks and bell pepper in a 13" × 9" baking dish. Add the broth, lemon juice, 2 teaspoons of the oil, thyme, and black pepper. Cover with foil and bake for 15 minutes.

Add the squash, olives, and salmon to the baking dish and drizzle with the remaining 1 teaspoon oil. Cover and bake for 30 minutes, or until the salmon is opaque and the vegetables are tender.

Place the penne in a large serving bowl. Break the salmon into bite-size pieces and add to the penne with the vegetables.

Makes 6 servings
Per serving: 402 calories, 7 g total fat, 1 g saturated fat, 21 mg cholesterol, 5 g dietary fiber, 121 mg sodium

Linguine with Clams
  12 ounces spinach linguine
  1 tablespoon olive oil
  2 shallots, chopped
  1 clove garlic, minced
  1 cup chopped plum tomatoes
  1 cup dry white wine or alcohol-free wine
  1 1/2 cups chicken broth

$^{1}/_{4}$ cup + 2 tablespoons chopped Italian parsley
3 dozen littleneck clams, scrubbed

Prepare the linguine according to package directions.

Meanwhile, in a large saucepot or Dutch oven heat the oil over medium-high heat. Add the shallots and garlic and cook, stirring often, for 4 minutes, or until soft. Add the tomatoes and cook for 1 minute. Add the wine and bring to a boil. Cook for 2 minutes. Add the broth and parsley. Bring to a boil.

Add the clams, cover, and cook for 5 minutes, or until the clams open. (Discard any unopened clams.)

Remove the clams to a bowl with a slotted spoon. Return the broth mixture to the heat and bring to a boil. Boil for 4 minutes, or until reduced by one-third. Remove 24 of the clams from their shells and mince; discard those shells. Keep the remaining 12 clams in their shells.

Add the minced clams and pasta to the pot. Toss to combine. Add the clams in the shells.

Makes 4 servings
Per serving: 312 calories, 6 g total fat, 1 g saturated fat, 76 mg cholesterol, 3 g dietary fiber, 425 mg sodium

Turkey and Bean Soft Tacos
8 corn tortillas (6" diameter)
8 ounces (2 cups) shredded cooked turkey breast
1 cup drained and rinsed canned kidney or pinto beans
1 $^{1}/_{4}$ cups mild or medium-spicy salsa + additional for topping
$^{1}/_{2}$ teaspoon ground cumin
1 $^{1}/_{2}$ cups finely shredded cabbage
1 large carrot, shredded
$^{1}/_{4}$ cup finely chopped sweet white onion
$^{1}/_{4}$ cup reduced-fat cucumber ranch dressing

Preheat the oven to 350°F.

Stack the tortillas and wrap them in foil. Place the tortillas in the oven and heat for 10 minutes.

Meanwhile, heat a large skillet coated with cooking spray over high heat. Add the turkey, beans, 1 1/4 cups of the salsa, and cumin and bring to a boil. Reduce the heat to low, cover, and simmer, stirring, for 10 minutes, or until heated through.

In a medium bowl, combine the cabbage, carrot, onion, and ranch dressing.

Spoon about 1/3 cup of the turkey filling into a tortilla. Top with 1/4 cup of the cabbage mixture and fold over. Repeat with the remaining tortillas, turkey filling, and cabbage mixture. Top with the remaining salsa.

Makes 4 servings

Per serving: 330 calories, 6 g total fat, 1 g saturated fat, 47 mg cholesterol, 8 g dietary fiber, 676 mg sodium

Turkey Meatloaf*

1 pound ground lean turkey
1/2 cup rolled oats
1 large egg
1 tablespoon dehydrated onion
1/2 cup ketchup

Preheat the oven to 350°F. Coat a loaf pan with cooking spray.

Combine the turkey, oats, egg, onion, and ketchup. Mix well and pack the mixture into the prepared loaf pan. Bake for 25 minutes, or until a thermometer inserted in the center registers 165°F and the meat is no longer pink.

Cut into five slices and serve.

Makes 5 servings

Per serving: 196 calories, 7 g total fat, 2 g saturated fat, 103 mg cholesterol, 1 g dietary fiber, 217 mg sodium

Chicken and Spanish Rice*

1 cup chopped onion
1/4 cup chopped green bell pepper
2 teaspoons vegetable oil
1 can (8 ounces) tomato sauce (see note)
1 teaspoon chopped fresh parsley
1/2 teaspoon freshly ground black pepper
1 1/4 teaspoons minced garlic
5 cups cooked rice
3 1/2 cups cooked, diced chicken breast

Heat the oil in a large skillet over medium heat. Add the onion and bell pepper and cook, stirring frequently, for 5 minutes, or until the vegetables start to soften. Add the tomato sauce, parsley, black pepper, and garlic. Heat through.

Add the cooked rice and chicken, and heat through.

Makes 5 servings
Per serving: 406 calories, 6 g total fat, 2 g saturated fat, 75 mg cholesterol, 2 g dietary fiber, 367 mg sodium
Health note: To reduce the sodium content of this recipe, use one 4-ounce can of no-salt-added tomato sauce and one 4-ounce can of regular tomato sauce.

Chicken Breasts Arrabbiata

1 tablespoon extra-virgin olive oil
1 large red bell pepper, chopped
1 large onion, chopped
1/4 cup seeded, rinsed, and chopped pepperoncini
3 cloves garlic, crushed
1 teaspoon dried basil, crushed
1/2 teaspoon freshly ground black pepper
1/4 teaspoon salt
3 cups coarsely chopped plum tomatoes
1/4 cup chicken broth

  1 tablespoon balsamic vinegar
  1 tablespoon tomato paste
  4 boneless, skinless chicken breast halves

In a large skillet, heat the oil over medium heat. Add the bell pepper, onion, pepperoncini, garlic, basil, black pepper, and salt. Cook, stirring, for 4 minutes, or until the vegetables are tender. Add the tomatoes, broth, vinegar, and tomato paste. Increase the heat to medium-high and cook, stirring, for 3 minutes, or until the tomatoes start to release their juices.

Add the chicken, reduce the heat to medium-low, cover, and simmer for 15 minutes, or until a thermometer inserted in the thickest portion registers 160°F and the juices run clear.

Makes 4 servings
Per serving: 225 calories, 6 g total fat, 1 g saturated fat, 66 mg cholesterol, 3 g dietary fiber, 491 mg sodium

Spicy Baked Fish*
  1 pound cod (or other fish) fillet
  1 tablespoon olive oil
  1 teaspoon salt-free spicy seasoning

Preheat the oven to 350°F. Coat a 9" × 9" baking dish with cooking spray.

Wash and dry the fish and place in the baking dish.

In a small bowl, combine the oil and seasoning. Drizzle over the fish.

Bake uncovered for 15 minutes or until the fish flakes with a fork. Cut into 4 pieces. Serve with rice.

Makes 4 servings
Per serving: 133 calories, 1 g total fat, 0 g saturated fat, 77 mg cholesterol, 0 g dietary fiber, 119 mg sodium

Orange Roughy Veracruz

4 orange roughy or red snapper fillets (5 ounces each)
1 tablespoon lime juice
1 teaspoon dried oregano, crushed
1 tablespoon olive oil
1 onion, chopped
1 clove garlic, minced
1 can (15 ounces) Mexican-style diced tomatoes
12 pimiento-stuffed olives, coarsely chopped
2 tablespoons chopped parsley

Preheat the oven to 350°F. Coat a 9" × 9" baking dish with cooking spray. Place the fillets in the baking dish. Sprinkle with the lime juice and oregano.

In a medium skillet, heat the oil over medium heat. Add the onion and garlic and cook, stirring occasionally, for 5 minutes, or until soft. Add the tomatoes (with juice), olives, and parsley. Cook, stirring occasionally, for 5 minutes, or until thickened. Spoon over the fillets. Cover tightly with foil.

Bake for 15 minutes, or until the fish flakes easily.

Makes 4 servings
Per serving: 185 calories, 6 g total fat, 1 g saturated fat, 28 mg cholesterol, 2 g dietary fiber, 510 mg sodium

Pan-Seared Red Snapper with Olive Crust

1⅓ cups fresh bread crumbs
¼ cup chopped fresh oregano, basil, or thyme
16 pitted and finely chopped kalamata olives
2 tablespoons freshly grated Parmesan cheese
½ teaspoon freshly ground black pepper
4 red snapper fillets (5 ounces each)

In a shallow bowl, combine the bread crumbs; oregano, basil, or thyme; olives; cheese; and pepper. Firmly press the fillets

into the mixture to coat evenly on both sides. Coat the top
of the fillets with cooking spray.

Heat a large cast-iron skillet coated with cooking spray
over medium-high heat. Add the fillets and cook, turning
once, for 6 minutes, or until the fish flakes easily.

Makes 4 servings

Per serving: 204 calories, 6 g total fat, 1 g saturated fat, 54
mg cholesterol, 1 g dietary fiber, 295 mg sodium

Cooking tip: Here's a quick sauce to serve with the fish. In a
food processor, combine 1 can (14½ ounces) stewed tomatoes, 1 tablespoon chopped fresh oregano, and 1 tablespoon balsamic vinegar. Process until the mixture is chunky.
Warm the sauce on the stove top or in the microwave.

Blackened Snapper

1 teaspoon paprika
½ teaspoon dried oregano, crushed
¼ teaspoon garlic powder
¼ teaspoon onion powder
¼ teaspoon salt
¼ teaspoon ground black pepper
⅛ teaspoon ground red pepper
4 red snapper fillets (5 ounces each)
2 teaspoons olive oil

In a small bowl, combine the paprika, oregano, garlic powder, onion powder, salt, black pepper, and red pepper.

Coat a large cast-iron skillet with cooking spray and heat
over high heat. Brush both sides of the snapper with the oil
and rub with the spice mixture. Place in the skillet and cook,
turning once, for 6 minutes, or until the fish flakes easily.

Makes 4 servings

Per serving: 175 calories, 6 g total fat, 1 g saturated fat, 53
mg cholesterol, 0 g dietary fiber, 266 mg sodium

Cooking tip: Almost any firm, white-fleshed fish can be used in this recipe. Try grouper, sea bass, redfish (red drum), or pompano in place of the snapper.

Five-Alarm Shrimp

1/4 cup cornstarch
1/2 teaspoon salt
1 pound jumbo shrimp, peeled and deveined
1 tablespoon canola oil
4 scallions, coarsely chopped
2 red or yellow bell peppers, cut into thin strips
2 tablespoons chopped fresh cilantro or parsley
2 cloves garlic, minced
1 serrano chile pepper, seeded and chopped (wear plastic
    gloves when handling)
1 tablespoon lime juice
3 tablespoons water
3/4 teaspoon crushed black peppercorns

In a shallow bowl, combine the cornstarch and salt. Add the shrimp and toss to coat well.

Heat the oil in a large nonstick skillet over medium-high heat. Add the shrimp and cook for 3 minutes, or until just opaque. Add the scallions, bell peppers, cilantro or parsley, garlic, and chile pepper and cook, stirring often, for 1 minute. Add the lime juice, water, and peppercorns. Cook, stirring constantly, for 1 minute, or until the shrimp are opaque.

Makes 4 servings
Per serving: 203 calories, 6 g total fat, 1 g saturated fat, 172 mg cholesterol, 2 g dietary fiber, 464 mg sodium

Shrimp with Chard and Red Beans

4 cloves garlic, minced
1 1/2 teaspoons paprika
1 teaspoon dried thyme, crushed
1/2 teaspoon freshly ground black pepper

¼ teaspoon salt

¼ teaspoon ground red pepper

1 pound large shrimp, peeled and deveined, tails left on

2 tablespoons olive oil

2 ribs celery, thinly sliced

1 large onion, chopped

1 large green bell pepper, chopped

¾ cup chicken broth

3 cups green or red Swiss chard, thinly sliced

1 can (14–19 ounces) red kidney beans

In a medium bowl, combine the garlic, paprika, thyme, black pepper, salt, and red pepper. Remove about half of the mixture to a small bowl. Add the shrimp to the medium bowl and toss to coat well.

Heat 1 tablespoon of the oil in a large saucepot or Dutch oven over medium heat. Add the celery, onion, and bell pepper. Cook, stirring frequently, for 6 minutes, or until crisp-tender.

Add the reserved spice mixture and cook, stirring frequently, for 2 minutes. Add ¼ cup of the broth. Cover and cook, stirring often, for 5 minutes.

Add the chard and cook, stirring frequently, for 2 minutes, or until wilted. Stir in the beans and the remaining ½ cup broth and bring to a boil over high heat. Reduce the heat to low, cover, and simmer for 10 minutes to blend the flavors.

Meanwhile, heat the remaining 1 tablespoon oil in a large skillet over high heat. Add the shrimp and cook, stirring occasionally, for 3 minutes, or until the shrimp are opaque.

Makes 4 servings

Per serving: 306 calories, 9 g total fat, 1 g saturated fat, 172 mg cholesterol, 9 g dietary fiber, 733 mg sodium

Tamale Pie

1 tablespoon olive oil

2 large red and/or green bell peppers, chopped

4–5 teaspoons chili powder

2 cans (14–19 ounces each) kidney beans, rinsed and drained

1 can (14½ ounces) diced tomatoes with green chiles

1 can (14½ ounces) diced tomatoes, drained

1 cup yellow cornmeal

¾ cup whole grain pastry flour

1 teaspoon baking powder

½ teaspoon baking soda

¼ teaspoon salt

1 cup (8 ounces) fat-free plain yogurt

1 cup (4 ounces) shredded reduced-fat Cheddar cheese

1 egg

2 tablespoons olive oil

Preheat the oven to 375°F. Coat an 11" × 7" baking dish with cooking spray.

Heat the oil in a large nonstick skillet over medium-high heat. Add the bell peppers and cook, stirring frequently, for 7 minutes, or until tender. Stir in the chili powder, beans, tomatoes with chiles, and diced tomatoes. Bring to a boil. Place in the prepared baking dish.

Meanwhile, in a large bowl, combine the cornmeal, flour, baking powder, baking soda, and salt. Add the yogurt, cheese, egg, and oil and combine just until blended.

Spoon the cornmeal mixture in spoonfuls over the filling, gently spreading it to cover. Place the baking dish on a baking sheet to catch any spillover.

Bake for 25 minutes, or until the crust is lightly browned and firm and the filling is bubbly.

Let stand for 10 minutes before serving.

Makes 6 servings

Per serving: 415 calories, 13 g total fat, 4 g saturated fat, 14 mg cholesterol, 13 g dietary fiber, 690 mg sodium

Spaghetti Squash Casserole

1 spaghetti squash, halved lengthwise and seeded
1 tablespoon vegetable oil
2 cloves garlic, chopped
1 small onion, chopped
1 teaspoon dried basil, crushed
2 plum tomatoes, chopped
8 ounces 1% cottage cheese
½ cup (2 ounces) shredded low-fat mozzarella cheese
¼ cup chopped parsley
¼ teaspoon salt
¼ cup (1 ounce) freshly grated Parmesan cheese
3 tablespoons seasoned dry bread crumbs

Preheat the oven to 400°F. Coat a 13" × 9" baking dish and a baking sheet with cooking spray.

Place the squash, cut side down, on the prepared baking sheet. Bake for 30 minutes, or until tender. With a fork, scrape the squash strands into a large bowl.

Meanwhile, in a medium skillet, heat the oil over medium heat. Add the garlic, onion, and basil and cook for 4 minutes, or until the onion is soft. Add the tomatoes and cook for 3 minutes, or until the mixture is dry.

To the bowl with the squash, add the cottage cheese, mozzarella, parsley, salt, and the tomato mixture. Toss to coat. Place in the prepared baking dish. Sprinkle with the Parmesan and bread crumbs.

Bake for 30 minutes, or until hot and bubbly.

Makes 6 servings

Per serving: 219 calories, 7 g total fat, 3 g saturated fat, 10 mg cholesterol, 4 g dietary fiber, 528 mg sodium

Cooking tip: Spaghetti squash can also be prepared in the

microwave oven. Pierce the squash in several places with a knife. Place on a microwaveable plate and cover loosely with a piece of plastic wrap. Cook on high power, turning twice, for 20 minutes, or until tender when pierced. Remove and let stand until cool enough to handle.

DESSERTS

Rich 'N Creamy Brown Rice Pudding

3 cups vanilla soy milk
1/2 cup uncooked brown rice
1/2 teaspoon salt
1/4 teaspoon freshly grated nutmeg
2 eggs, lightly beaten
1/2 cup dried cherries

In a medium saucepan, combine the milk, rice, salt, and nutmeg. Bring to a boil over high heat. Reduce the heat to low, cover, and simmer for 45 minutes. Remove from the heat and let cool for 5 minutes.

Stir 1/2 cup of the rice mixture into the eggs, stirring constantly. Gradually stir the egg mixture into the saucepan. Stir in the cherries.

Place over medium-low heat and cook, stirring constantly, for 5 minutes, or until thickened. Serve warm or refrigerate to serve cold later.

Makes 4 servings
Per serving: 242 calories, 7 g total fat, 1 g saturated fat, 106 mg cholesterol, 3 g dietary fiber, 347 mg sodium

Broiled Peaches and Strawberries

5 medium peaches, cut into 1" wedges
1 1/2 pints strawberries, hulled and quartered
2 tablespoons honey
1/2 teaspoon ground cinnamon

⅛ teaspoon ground allspice or cloves

1 tablespoon butter, cut into small pieces

3 tablespoons slivered fresh mint, lemon verbena, or cinnamon basil (optional)

Preheat the broiler. Coat a large baking sheet with sides with cooking spray.

In a large bowl, combine the peaches, strawberries, honey, cinnamon, and allspice or cloves and toss to coat well. Place the fruit on the prepared baking sheet. Dot with the butter.

Broil, turning the pan 2 or 3 times (no need to turn the fruit), for 4 minutes, or until the fruit is glazed, bubbly, and golden brown in spots. Remove from the oven and let cool slightly.

Sprinkle with the mint, lemon verbena, or cinnamon basil, if using. Serve warm or at room temperature.

Makes 6 servings

Per serving: 111 calories, 3 g total fat, 1 g saturated fat, 5 mg cholesterol, 4 g dietary fiber, 23 mg sodium

Pear and Almond Crisp

4 large pears, cored and sliced ½" thick

2 tablespoons maple syrup

1 tablespoon lemon juice

1 teaspoon vanilla extract

½ teaspoon freshly grated nutmeg

1 cup rolled oats (not quick-cooking)

⅓ cup sliced natural almonds

¼ cup packed brown sugar

2 tablespoons whole grain pastry flour

2 tablespoons cold butter, cut into small pieces

2 tablespoons canola oil

Preheat the oven to 350°F.

Combine the pears, maple syrup, lemon juice, vanilla extract, and nutmeg in an 11" × 7" baking dish.

In a medium bowl, combine the oats, almonds, brown sugar, flour, butter, and oil and mix with your fingers to form crumbs. Sprinkle the topping over the pear mixture.

Bake for 40 minutes, or until the pears are tender and bubbly and the topping is lightly browned.

Makes 8 servings

Per serving: 271 calories, 10 g total fat, 3 g saturated fat, 8 mg cholesterol, 5 g dietary fiber, 134 mg sodium

Strawberry Tart with Oat-Cinnamon Crust
Crust
⅔ cup rolled oats
½ cup whole grain pastry flour
1 tablespoon sugar
1 teaspoon ground cinnamon
¼ teaspoon baking soda
2 tablespoons canola oil
2–3 tablespoons fat-free plain yogurt

Filling
¼ cup strawberry all-fruit spread
½ teaspoon vanilla extract
1½ pints strawberries, hulled

To make the crust: Preheat the oven to 375°F. Coat a baking sheet with cooking spray.

In a medium bowl, combine the oats, flour, sugar, cinnamon, and baking soda. Stir in the oil and 2 tablespoons of the yogurt to make a soft, slightly sticky dough. If the dough is too stiff, add the remaining 1 tablespoon yogurt.

Place the dough on the prepared baking sheet and pat evenly into a 10" circle. If the dough sticks to your hands, coat them lightly with cooking spray.

Place a 9" cake pan on the dough and trace around it with a sharp knife. With your fingers, push up and pinch the dough around the outside of the circle to make a 9" circle with a rim ¼" high.

Bake for 15 minutes, or until firm and golden. Remove from the oven and set aside to cool.

To make the filling: Meanwhile, in a small microwaveable bowl, combine the all-fruit spread and vanilla extract. Microwave on high power for 10 to 15 seconds, or until melted.

Brush a generous tablespoon evenly over the cooled crust. Arrange the strawberries evenly over the crust. Brush the remaining spread evenly over the strawberries, making sure to get some of the spread between the strawberries to secure them.

Refrigerate for at least 30 minutes, or until the spread has jelled.

Makes 6 servings

Per serving: 187 calories, 6 g total fat, 0 g saturated fat, 0 mg cholesterol, 3 g dietary fiber, 65 mg sodium

Cooking tip: For a calcium boost, you can serve the tart with a scoop of fat-free vanilla frozen yogurt on the side.

Apple Crumble with Toasted-Oat Topping

6 medium Jonagold or Golden Delicious apples, cored and thinly sliced (see note)

½ cup unsweetened applesauce

¾ cup rolled oats

3 tablespoons toasted wheat germ

3 tablespoons packed light brown sugar

1 teaspoon ground cinnamon

1 tablespoon canola oil

1 tablespoon unsalted butter, cut into small pieces

Preheat the oven to 350°F. Coat a 13" × 9" baking dish with cooking spray.

Combine the apples and applesauce in the prepared baking dish.

In a small bowl, combine the oats, wheat germ, brown sugar, and cinnamon. Add the oil and butter. Mix with your fingers to form crumbs. Sprinkle the oat mixture evenly over the apples.

Bake for 30 minutes, or until the topping is golden and the apples are bubbling.

Makes 6 servings

Per serving: 207 calories, 6 g total fat, 2 g saturated fat, 5 mg cholesterol, 6 g dietary fiber, 3 mg sodium

Cooking tip: Although you can make this recipe with peeled apples, leaving the peels on ensures that you get more fiber as well as the beneficial antioxidant quercetin.

Olive Oil–Cornmeal Cake with Blueberry and Red Wine Sauce

Cake

1 cup yellow cornmeal

¾ cup sugar

½ cup whole grain pastry flour

1¼ teaspoons baking powder

½ teaspoon baking soda

¼ teaspoon salt

2 eggs

2 egg whites

½ cup (4 ounces) fat-free plain yogurt

¼ cup extra-virgin olive oil

1 tablespoon freshly grated orange peel

2 tablespoons orange juice

1 tablespoon confectioners' sugar (optional)

Sauce

1 pint fresh or frozen blueberries
¼ cup dry red wine
1 tablespoon orange juice
Pinch of ground nutmeg

To make the cake: Preheat the oven to 350°F. Coat an 8" round cake pan with cooking spray. Line the pan bottom with a round of waxed paper and coat the waxed paper with cooking spray.

In a large bowl, combine the cornmeal, sugar, flour, baking powder, baking soda, and salt.

In a medium bowl, using a wire whisk, beat the eggs, egg whites, yogurt, oil, orange peel, and orange juice. (The mixture may look curdled.) Add to the cornmeal mixture and stir just until blended. Place in the prepared pan.

Bake for 25 minutes, or until browned, firm, and a wooden pick inserted off-center comes out clean.

Cool in the pan on a rack for 30 minutes. Loosen the edges and turn the cake out onto the rack. Peel off the waxed paper and let cool completely.

To make the sauce: In a medium saucepan, combine the blueberries, wine, orange juice, and nutmeg. Bring to a boil over medium-high heat, stirring constantly. Boil for 1 minute.

Reduce the heat to low, cover, and simmer, stirring frequently, for 5 minutes, or until the blueberries are tender and the sauce is thickened.

Place the sauce in a bowl, partially cover, and let cool. Dust the cake with confectioners' sugar, if using, and serve with the sauce.

Makes 8 servings

Per serving: 274 calories, 9 g total fat, 1 g saturated fat, 53 mg cholesterol, 3 g dietary fiber, 263 mg sodium

Carrot Cake with Cream Cheese Frosting
Cake

2 cups whole grain pastry flour

2 teaspoons baking powder

2 teaspoons baking soda

1 teaspoon ground cinnamon

1/4 teaspoon salt

1 cup granulated sugar

2 eggs

2 egg whites

1/3 cup canola oil

2 teaspoons vanilla extract

1 cup buttermilk or fat-free plain yogurt (see note)

2 cups finely shredded carrots

1/2 cup golden raisins

1/2 cup well-drained crushed pineapple

Frosting

2 ounces reduced-fat cream cheese, at room temperature

2 tablespoons unsalted butter, at room temperature

1 1/4 cups confectioners' sugar

1/2 teaspoon vanilla extract

3 tablespoons chopped walnuts or pecans

To make the cake: Preheat the oven to 350°F. Coat two 8" round cake pans with cooking spray.

In a medium bowl, combine the flour, baking powder, baking soda, cinnamon, and salt.

In a large bowl, using a wire whisk, beat the granulated sugar, eggs, egg whites, oil, and vanilla extract until well-blended and frothy. Whisk in the buttermilk or yogurt. Stir in the carrots, raisins, and pineapple. Add the flour mixture and stir just until blended.

Evenly divide the batter between the prepared cake pans.

Bake for 25 minutes, or until a wooden pick inserted in the center comes out clean.

Cool the cakes in the pans on racks for 30 minutes. Loosen the edges and turn the cakes out onto the racks to cool completely.

To make the frosting: In a medium bowl, with an electric mixer on medium-high speed, beat the cream cheese and butter just until blended. Beat in the confectioners' sugar and vanilla extract until light and fluffy.

Place one cake layer on a plate. Spread the top of the layer with frosting, but not the sides. Place the other cake layer on top. Spread the top of the layer with the remaining frosting. Sprinkle with the walnuts or pecans.

Makes 10 servings

Per serving: 445 calories, 13 g total fat, 3 g saturated fat, 53 mg cholesterol, 4 g dietary fiber, 467 mg sodium

Cooking tip: If you don't have buttermilk or yogurt, you can use soured milk instead. To make soured milk, pour the desired amount of 1% milk into a measuring cup. Add 1 tablespoon lemon juice or cider vinegar. Let stand for 10 minutes.

PART V

Real-Life Secrets to Beat High Blood Pressure

Fencing Broke Down His Fitness Barrier

At the tender age of 21, Dan Collins was so overweight and out of shape that his doctor feared he was killing himself. "I was 5 foot 10½ and weighed 239 pounds," Dan says. "I was diagnosed with high blood pressure, and my doctor was concerned enough to put me on medication."

That was in 1984. Rather than sit back and let medication take control of his life, the young newspaper reporter from Towson, Maryland, embarked on a complete body makeover. He dramatically reduced the amount of salt in his diet, put the brakes on his runaway eating habits, and began riding a stationary bike and walking on a regular basis.

Two years later, Dan had reined in his blood pressure and was down to a lean 182 pounds. He felt and looked great. But he feared that he was entering an exercise slump. "I didn't mind the walking and other activities, but I wanted a different kind of sport that I really could get into," he says. "I knew that was important if I was going to keep off the weight for good."

Back then, everyone seemed to be doing aerobics à

la Jane Fonda. But Dan opted for a less trendy sport: fencing. Each time he donned his mask and protective vest and picked up his foil, his workouts seemed more fun and exciting. That's because fencing is both physically and mentally demanding. "Few people realize that a good fencer needs both aerobic and anaerobic conditioning as well as a sense of strategy and emotional control," says Dan, who's cofounder of the Chesapeake Fencing Club of Baltimore.

Many a basement and attic has an assortment of sports gear that's collecting dust from years of nonuse. But not Dan's. He continues to fence every week, just as he s for the past 17 years. He also works out at home u a stationary bike and free weights to enhance his fen performance. It seems this lean, mean fencing maci has found the perfect activity to help him stay trim in control of his blood pressure.

TAKE-HOME ADVICE

Go for the unusual and exotic. If you are hav g a hard time sticking with a workout regimen, try an uncommon or unconventional activity, like African dance, tai chi, or scuba diving. Part of the journey of getting in shape—an important component of any blood pressure–management plan—is discovering the real you. Let your workouts be an expression of your inner self.

She Got the Support
She Needed

At age 29, Olivia Williamson learned that she had high blood pressure. Her doctor told her that unless she did something about it, Olivia could be on medication for the rest of her life.

Olivia knew what that "something" was. After all, she weighed 240 pounds. "I had no choice but to slim down," she says. "Having high blood pressure really scared me."

It's not that Olivia hadn't tried to lose weight before. She was no stranger to diet-and-exercise regimens. But she could never stick with them on her own. This time, she decided, she'd enlist help.

Luckily for Olivia, her employer, Stanford University, offers a 6-week weight-management course through the school's medical center. Once the class is over, students can attend weekly support-group meetings for up to 4 months. Olivia signed on.

For the first 10 weeks, she diligently followed the directions of the class instructor, cutting back on fat, eating less in one sitting, and exercising moderately. But she didn't lose a single pound. Was she frustrated? You bet. But the support group kept Olivia going.

"Just being able to tell the group, 'I'm doing it, I'm sticking with it,' made me feel better," says Olivia, of Mountain View, California. "It allowed me to settle into the healthier habits that I was learning." She enjoyed the group so much that when her weight-management course ended, she joined an e-mail diet-support network that she found through Stanford.

Within a year, Olivia lost 45 pounds, and her blood pressure returned to a healthy level. As a bonus, she had more energy than ever before, which encouraged her to stay active in her daily life. "When I went on a sightseeing trip to Europe in 1999, I was able to climb all 380 steps to the top of Notre-Dame Cathedral," she says. "I wouldn't have been able to do that before!"

TAKE-HOME ADVICE

Seek out support. In a support group, you meet people who are facing the same challenges as you. It's a perfect forum for exchanging advice on what works and what doesn't, for unloading your frustrations, and for celebrating your victories. To locate a support group near you, start by contacting local hospitals and churches. Look in the blue pages of your phone book, under "Self-Help Support Groups." Or check to see if your employer keeps a list of local resources.

Her Small Changes Made a Huge Difference

A routine visit to the doctor totally changed Tammy Munson's life.

Tammy, a resident of Jamestown, New York, admits that she knew very little about good nutrition when she was younger. She routinely ate high-fat foods such as Buffalo wings, pepperoni pizza, and french fries—and she couldn't understand why she kept gaining weight. "I just didn't know any better," she says. By age 21, she weighed 253 pounds.

Then, during a routine checkup, Tammy found out that she had alarmingly high blood pressure. The news jolted her into action. Determined to slim down, she began paying more attention to her diet. She switched from 2% milk and regular soft drinks to fat-free milk and diet soft drinks—and lost 30 pounds. She had never considered how her beverage choices contributed to her calorie intake. This surprised her so much that she decided to learn everything she could about healthy eating.

"I went to the library and signed out every nutrition book I could find," she says. "I was determined to make better food choices so that I could lose more weight."

She also read dozens of cookbooks and discovered how to turn fat-laden recipes into nutritious meals with a few simple ingredient substitutions.

All of that reading transformed Tammy's eating habits. Within about a year, she lost a total of 147 pounds. And she has stayed at 106 pounds ever since, thanks to her attention and commitment to good nutrition.

TAKE-HOME ADVICE

Find out what you're really eating. For one day, write down everything that you eat and drink, along with the fat and calorie content of each item. At the end of the day, add up your numbers. Surprise! You're probably eating more than you realized, which could be expanding your waistline—and raising your blood pressure to boot.

She Slimmed Down by Keeping Up with Her Grandchild

Dolly Higgins's slow-speed life—and metabolism—cranked up several notches once she started chasing her granddaughter.

When seventy-year-old Dolly retired, her lifestyle took a turn for the worse. The Boston grandmother found herself sleeping and eating a lot. Soon, she weighed 170 pounds, far too much for her 5-foot-2-inch frame. The excess weight pressed on a herniated disk in her back, leaving her bed-bound for weeks. Then she found out that she had high blood pressure and borderline diabetes.

Dolly knew that her weight had contributed to her health problems. She also knew that she needed to dump those excess pounds. But she couldn't get herself started. A favor for her daughter turned out to be the boost she needed.

"My daughter had taken a third job and needed me to help watch Alisha, my granddaughter," Dolly explains. "I was thrilled. I needed a reason to get out of bed every morning."

On fair-weather days, Dolly walked Alisha to school in the morning and then returned to pick her up in the afternoon. When Dolly took Alisha to the local pool twice a week, she did some swimming herself. She also started swimming at the YMCA on "senior days." As Alisha got older, Dolly joined her for bike rides, an activity she enjoyed so much that she even bought a stationary bike for winter.

During the first year and a half, Dolly lost 40 pounds, going from a size 18 to 10. Today, she feels great and has an excellent health record. Though she no longer watches her granddaughter as often, Dolly has maintained her new, active lifestyle.

TAKE-HOME ADVICE

Keep up with a kid. If you don't have children or grandchildren of your own to chase around, make friends with youngsters in your neighborhood. Or volunteer to help out at a nearby day-care center or elementary school. Kids have so much energy that keeping up with them is a challenge. But you can sure have a blast—and burn some calories—trying. Who says losing weight and lowering your blood pressure can't be fun?

She's Getting the Upper Hand on Stress

In retrospect, Brita Hudson-Smith isn't surprised that her blood pressure rose to 140/90. When she found out about it in her early thirties, she was under considerable stress as she coped with the death of her mother. Even before that, she had been gaining weight. And she had a family history of high blood pressure.

At the time, however, Brita was shocked to find out that her blood pressure had climbed so high. "You don't really pay attention to your risks until they lead to a bigger problem," she says.

Her doctor put her on high blood pressure medication right away. But she didn't work very hard at making basic lifestyle changes until a few years later, when she left her high-stress job at a health organization in suburban Philadelphia.

"I started walking every day," Brita says. "I got involved in my community, and I read books about health and spirituality. I also meditated every day and became a vegetarian. It took time, but my blood pressure went down even further."

But the changes didn't last. When Brita started a new

job the following year, her health routine fell apart. Her blood pressure rose higher than it had ever been. At one point, it reached an alarming 170/100. That landed her in the hospital.

Now in her fifties, Brita admits that she still struggles to find a balance between career demands and healthful living. "I keep saying a mantra to myself: 'I'm not going to let my job keep me from eating right and exercising.' "

She continues to take medication, but she also eases daily stress by visiting friends and doing things she enjoys, like flower arranging and going to the theater. "I know that I don't have to do everything, that letting go of some things is okay," she says. "I write little notes to myself about the priorities in my life. I read them whenever my life gets a little crazy."

TAKE-HOME ADVICE

Schedule relaxation into your day. A little stress can be a good thing. But too much for too long can raise your risk of a heart attack—especially if you also have high blood pressure as a risk factor. What's more, stress can contribute to unhealthy eating habits, which can aggravate high blood pressure even more. So no matter how busy you are, make time to unwind. Even 10 minutes of walking or deep breathing can defuse your body's stress response.

Variety Spices Up
Her Workouts

Whenever Cheryl Allard goes to the gym, she abides by her 10-minute rule: Use one machine for 10 minutes, then move on to something else. This strategy helped her beat the boredom that nearly ended her exercise program. It also helped her lose 100 pounds.

Cheryl began working out in 1997 after finding out that she had high blood pressure. At the time, she weighed 265 pounds.

"I was chubby even as a child," recalls the sewing machine consultant from Chicago. "My parents lived in England during World War II, when food was rationed. They had the mindset that food was never to be wasted. I was raised to clean my plate."

As Cheryl got older, the pounds kept piling on. "I tried every diet under the sun to slim down," she says. "Once, I even lost 40 pounds, but they all came back."

Then, Cheryl's husband persuaded her to get a physical. "I hadn't been to our family doctor in years, and my husband kept bugging me to go," she explains. "I went just to keep him quiet."

But Cheryl was the one left speechless after her doctor

handed her a prescription for blood pressure medication. "That got me motivated to lose," she says. "I didn't want to be taking pills for the rest of my life."

Cheryl went to a nutrition counselor, who helped her revamp her eating habits. She also joined a local gym, where she started using the aerobic-exercise equipment. "I felt self-conscious at first, because of my size," she says.

Over time, her self-confidence grew—as did her boredom. Even though she varied her workouts, they seemed to drag on and on. But she knew that she couldn't stop exercising.

So she decided to add some variety to her workout routine. Rather than spending all of her time on one piece of equipment, she'd stay on for just 10 minutes, then switch. "I can do anything for 10 minutes," she says. "Even though I detest riding that bike, I do it, knowing that it's going to be for only 10 minutes." Usually, she ends up using four or five different machines.

That did the trick. Cheryl found herself looking forward to her workouts so much that she started going to the gym 6 days a week. Within a year of launching her weight-loss program, she took off 100 pounds.

In the years since, Cheryl has continued to eat sensibly and exercise regularly. And it shows: Her weight has held steady at 165 pounds. Even better, her blood pressure has returned to a healthy level, and she was able to stop taking her medication.

"When my son got married not too long ago, my relatives flew in from England," she says. "They were commenting on how much weight I had lost and how good I look. More important to me, though, is that I feel great!"

TAKE-HOME ADVICE

Go for 10, then switch. Cheryl is doing what the experts call circuit training, and it has more benefits than just beating boredom. By using different machines, you work different muscles, trimming and toning your entire body. And that helps melt away any extra pounds that may be contributing to your high blood pressure. You can ask a personal trainer to create a circuit for you, or you can come up with your own, as Cheryl did. Use treadmills, elliptical trainers, upright and recumbent bikes, stairclimbers, rowers—whatever aerobic machines your gym has available. Stay on one machine for 10 minutes, then move on to the next.

INDEX

**Eat Peanut Butter Every Day and Lose
All the Weight You Want!**

The Peanut Butter Diet

Holly McCord, M.A., R.D.
Nutrition Editor, *Prevention* Magazine

Recipe Coordinator, Regina Ragone, M.S., R.D.,
Food Editor, *Prevention* Magazine

You *can* eat peanut butter every day and still lose weight!
Many health-conscious dieters have shied away from this
tempting treat, but new studies show that peanut butter
can actually lower your risk for heart disease and diabetes
and help you shed unwanted pounds. And because THE
PEANUT BUTTER DIET is so satisfying, those who follow it are more successful at slimming down than those
who choose a traditional low-fat diet:

Dig in and discover:

- *50 fast-and-fabulous recipes*
- *4 weeks of delicious, super-easy meal
  plans*
- *A day-by-day diet you can stick to—even
  when you're eating out*
- *Fitness strategies to boost your
  metabolism and decrease body fat*
- *Special tips and treats for the whole
  family*

**AVAILABLE WHEREVER BOOKS ARE SOLD FROM
ST. MARTIN'S PAPERBACKS**

PNUT 5/02